THE WOMAN WHO LOST HER SKIN

THE WOMAN WHO LOST HER SKIN

(AND OTHER DERMATOLOGICAL TALES)

Dr Robert A. Norman

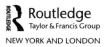
Routledge
Taylor & Francis Group

NEW YORK AND LONDON

First published 2004
by Routledge
11 New Fetter lane, London EC4P 4EE

Simultaneously published in the USA and Canada
by Routledge
29 West 35th Street, New York, NY 10001

Routledge is an imprint of the Taylor & Francis Group

Typeset in Times by Taylor & Francis
Printed and bound in Great Britain by The Cromwell Press Ltd.

British Library Cataloguing in Publication Data
A catalogue record for this book is available from the British Library

Library of Congress Cataloging in Publication Data
A catalog record for this book has been requested

ISBN 0-415-34356-9

CONTENTS

Dr Rob Norman's first job was as a caddy at Cascade Country Club in his hometown of Grand Rapids, Michigan. His next career move (at age 15) was to assist in the toy department at Herpolsheimer's, a huge downtown department store. Rob was quickly promoted to run the Christmas train attached to the ceiling of the bargain basement, 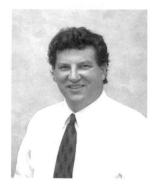 where mothers handed him rolls of dimes to keep their children on the train while they went shopping. It was at that time that he developed his first comedy act, keeping the kids entertained with jokes ("Did you hear the one about the mother who left her little kid on the train?") It was also at that point that he spent time soul-searching (almost ten minutes) and realized that retail was not his passion. He put his youthful efforts into medicine and writing.

He became an emergency room doc and family practitioner, and spent time in the Big Apple and Beantown, having his plays produced, and wrote a piece for the Letterman show. The opportunity came to be a dermatologic physician and surgeon and he grabbed it by the epidermis. Rob is a clinical instructor for several medical schools and has volunteered on medical committees to improve patient care. He participated in medical programs in Scotland, Haiti, and, in the fall of 2001, in Cuba. Rob has written 15 books, over 200 medical and general articles, including articles for *Discover* magazine. He wrote the lyrics, co-produced and played harmonica on two Blues CDs and continues to write comedy.

He and his wife Carol have five children. He knows none of them by first name but keeps pictures of them in his wallet so he can keep track when they ask for money.

ACKNOWLEDGEMENTS

Thanks to Karen Bowler and Claire Gauler of Routledge, London, for their incredible work. Much love to my wife Carol, my children and other family, my fellow doctors, students, office staff, and my patients. (Patients' stories have been adapted for this book and names and personal details have been changed.)

Chapters Two, Three and Five have previously been published in earlier forms in *Discover Magazine*; Chapter Four in an earlier form in *Cutis* magazine. Chapters One and Sixteen have been published in a book by Rob Norman – *Take Two Aspirin and See Yourself in the Morning* (Mancorp Publishing, 1997), and Chapter Five was published in *Mother Nature, Father Time* (North Shore Press, 1998).

ACKNOWLEDGEMENTS

FOREWORD

In this fascinating, delightful, insightful and informative account of frontline medicine Dr Robert Norman joins a notable list of physician storytellers who report their daily, intimate experiences for the enlightenment and entertainment of the public. He is a worthy descendant of the likes of Chekhov who brought the physician's eye to the comedies and tragedies of the sick and scared.

While this book is eminently readable and therefore susceptible to the criticism of being superficial – even funny – no one should be deceived by Norman's lively, narrative style. Chronic skin diseases cause a lot of misery with devastating effects on the quality of people's lives. Norman shows his empathetic skills in his humanistic, non-affected manner of cheerfully helping these patients.

Dr Norman is a scholar who possesses the rare ability to use the conversational form to communicate how the caring, compassionate doctor deals with frightened patients. He is the holistic doctor who takes into account patients' beliefs and feelings to the enhancement of a favorable therapeutic outcome.

Norman is a talking–listening doctor who knows how to avoid doctor-speak to learn more about his patients' fears and hopes. This book allows you become a close observer of what is actually going on in the patient–doctor encounter. Medical students, drowning in a Niagara of new evidence-based medicine, would do well to read this account. They will learn much more about the art of medicine than the professoriate has the time or interest to teach them.

In a time when doctors are widely thought to be merely technocrats who dispense medicines rather than psychological support and counseling, Norman's chatty account is an inspiration for those who long for that endangered species – the old-fashioned family doctor with a wonderful bedside manner, who instinctively knew more about healing than the molecular biologists of today. Moreover, by reading this book, harried doctors of today, threatened with a chaotic legal system and the bureaucratic hassles of managed care, can arm themselves against early bum-out and despair by seeing first-hand the satisfaction and joy that Norman gamers from his unique down-home style in fulfilling the Hippocratic goal of relieving suffering.

One further message of this richly textured, multi-layered saga is noteworthy, namely, you don't have to commit social suicide by becoming a doctor holed up in professional isolation from the beautiful outside world. Norman is a role model of balance in seeking the good life. You can raise five kids, be a sports enthusiast, engage in a wide range of community efforts and have a helluva lot of fun at the same time.

Albert Kligman, MD

One

LIQUID AIR

Since I'm a dermatologist, I need to give you the low-down on the skin. It's the body's largest organ, and truly an amazing structure. At twenty square feet and nine pounds, it's an excellent device to protect the inner environment.

The skin has three major components: the epidermis, dermis, and subcutaneous layers. The epidermis, the outermost layer of skin, has a top layer called the stratum corneum, composed of closely-packed cells which helps protect the skin from external abuse. Underneath are pigment cells, which provide our variation in color, and immune cells, which filter out foreign materials and dangerous substances. The middle layer is the dermis, where collagen, blood vessels, nerves, and other substrates live. Below the dermis is the fatty subcutaneous layer, which protects and insulates.

When you're a baby, your skin is elastic and resilient, and it changes every day from then on. We lose about 1% of collagen every year after age thirty, as well as elastic fibers and blood vessels that attach to the epidermis. The result is crinkles and wrinkles – a rather unfair exchange. The skin becomes sallow and pale. We increase fat deposition in the areas we don't like, and we lose fat and therefore insulation in other body areas such as the face, arms, and legs, which decreases our tolerance for cold. The underlying tissue depletion makes us more prone to injury, and the loss of nerves provides for poor heat tolerance.

Now, on top of all these natural occurrences of aging, consider increased exposure to UV light, alcohol, smoking, diet, and heredity. The protective ozone layer is thinning, and skin cancer rates are increasing. In the United States one person dies every hour from skin cancer; one third of all cancers are skin cancer, and 40-50% of all Americans who reach age 65 will develop skin cancer in their lifetime. And in the UK it is the fastest-growing and most common form of cancer, and skin cancer rates have doubled over the last 10 years, with over 40,000 new cases diagnosed each year.

Three basic types of skin cancer exist. The most common is basal cell, but this is also the least likely to spread. One third of all basal cells occur around the nose. Other common areas are on and around the ears, upper back, neck, and cheeks. Squamous cell cancers are more likely to spread, and, like basal cells, are generally the result of chronic sun exposure. Melanomas are the deadliest cancer. When a melanoma has grown to the size of a dime, it already has a 50% chance of having spread. The rate of melanoma in the US has doubled in the past 30 years and, each year, 53,600 people learn they have melanoma.

So how can we prevent these cancers from growing and killing?

Children must be protected from harmful exposure to UV rays. Studies have shown that the risk of developing skin cancer increases if they have three blistering sunburns before the age of 18. The younger a child is when the burns occur, the greater the risk.

I recommend every year on your birthday to get your birthday suit checked. Stay out of the sun, use sun blocks with a sun protection factor of 15 or greater every day, and use mild antibacterial soaps and cleansers. You should wear sunglasses with ultraviolet protective coating, and hats with brims wide enough to protect the head, ears, and neck. Special clothing can be purchased which protects the skin from UV damage. And remember, the UV light from tanning beds is equally dangerous. There is no such thing as a safe and glowing tan, unless one uses self-tanning creams. And remember that many medicines taken internally, such as

tetracycline and estrogens can increase sensitivity to
ultraviolet light and the chance of you burning your skin.

Many techniques are available for treatment of
cancerous and pre-cancerous lesions. Cryosurgery, the use of
liquid nitrogen for treatment of abnormal skin lesions, has
been used since the early 1900s. Whitehouse had an article
published in the *Journal of the American Medical
Association* in 1907 entitled "Liquid air in dermatology: its
indications and limitations." A doctor named Torre came
along in the 1960s and developed a practical apparatus to
use liquid air in a spray form. It rapidly developed into the
preferred method of cryosurgery for treating benign and
malignant lesions. When I ask my nurse if my guns are
loaded, she knows that I'm referring to the canisters I use to
administer my liquid nitrogen therapy. And, like many
dermatologists, I shoot them all day long.

When you think of it, liquid nitrogen is truly remarkable
– using liquid at sub-zero temperatures to destroy tissue in a
relatively easy manner. Destruction of malignant cells
requires a temperature at least as cold as -50 degrees
centigrade. Not only does it seem magical to me that the
liquid stays liquid at these temperatures, but the results can
be amazing.

How does it work? Cryosurgery targets the dermal–
epidermal junction providing separation and removal of
epidermal lesions. In simple terms, the nasty, unwanted
growths usually blister and fall off. And here are some of the
benefits compared to other surgery: very little, if any,
bleeding; no additional anesthesia is required; low rate of
wound infection; no sutures; a biopsy can be done while the
lesion is frozen; rapid healing; fast, easy procedure. Not bad.

The skin is an amazing, versatile organ. There are good
treatments available for your skin ills. My advice, however,
is to protect your skin and prevent skin cancers and other
problems. But you can always just mail me your stories.

Two

THE WOMAN WHO LOST HER SKIN

I was called to the hospital for a consult on a woman who my friend and fellow physician, Bill Cook, said he had admitted because she was "losing her skin." Bill was the primary care doctor for the 28-year-old woman, named Mary. He told me she had come to his office with the sudden onset of skin peeling, weakness, and painful and irritated eyes and mouth. From his description, I had an idea of Mary's disease, and made my way to see her prior to my morning office hours.

Hospitals are progressing to become more and more places of super-specialization, in which doctors trained strictly in hospital medicine ("hospitalists") will rule the domain. Most patients will be taken care of in sub-acute and outpatient settings, and only those in more critical conditions will roost in hospitals.

Before going in to see Mary, I reviewed her chart. She had been hospitalized the day before, and the routine admission orders such as chest x-ray and blood tests were in place. In addition, she had been placed on intravenous fluid replacement therapy and pain medications.

I found Mary in her bed, staring blankly up at the passing images on the TV. After approaching her side, I introduced myself. She smiled and said, "Hey."

"I'd like to take a look at your skin," I said. "If that's OK."

"What's left of it," she offered.

"I'll be back shortly," I said. I went out and found a nurse to help. A perky middle-aged woman named Peggy came to my aid. We both gloved, and she gently pulled back Mary's sheets. I tried to keep my most deadpan, yet alert, expression as I witnessed the devastation brought on by her disease. 'She may be looking right at me,' I thought, and I didn't want to add panic. An underlying blanket of red covered her entire skin surface, and the top layer was sloughing off in large sheets like wet wallpaper. Mary's face, neck, trunk, legs, feet – everywhere – had been captured by this crimson devil which appeared ready to take her down forever. I looked at the few islands of normal skin like a capsized sailor seeking refuge from a sea of fire. I had seen two other patients with this disorder before, but neither of this severity. What devastation!

I examined her everywhere – skin, genitals, mouth, and eyes – and then I pulled off my gloves. I looked up at Mary, who in fact was peering at me like a hunting dog who had found her prey. Peggy stood patiently by.

"Whaddayathink, Doc?" she asked. Her words slid together like a multiflavored ice cream cone that had melted. Apparently, she was groggy from her pain medications.

"It appears that you have a fairly severe reaction to a medicine you took," I said. "It doesn't happen very often, but when it does, it can be a real challenge. Here's the good news. I'm going to make sure you get the best treatment we have, and I'll let you know everything I recommend, OK?"

She nodded. "What happened?"

"Good question," I said. "Have you had medicines in the last few weeks?"

"I take something for my knees. It's like a pain pill, but it never gave me a problem before."

"Anything else?"

She pondered for a moment, her eyes focusing somewhere in the middle ground. "I did have an ear ache, and I took something I found in my cabinet. I'd have to check it. I remember one of the kids or somebody used it when they had an infection and it helped them, so I took it a few days."

"How long ago did you take it?" I queried.

"I think it was about two weeks ago," she said.

"And this just started a day or two ago?" I asked.

"Day before yesterday, yeah, I started losing my skin. Felt hot all over, and sick to my stomach. First I just had the rash on my face, arms and legs, and then it was all over, even my lips and my eyes. I got these blisters like I was in one of those horror movies after a nuclear explosion."

"Can you have the medicine brought here?" I asked.

"Sure," she said.

"Are you in much pain?" I asked.

"Not really. I feel kind of stoned," she said. "But I'm trying to take in everything you're telling me."

"The pain medications can make you feel quite tired," I said. "I appreciate the fact that you are trying to talk with me; it will definitely help in your care."

Stop for a moment. Can you imagine this? Do you remember the last time, if you have had a minor burn, you watched as a small part of your skin peeled off? Picture what it must be like if your entire skin peeled off. How would you feel about yourself? Imagine Mary the day before her skin rebellion, brushing her hair, putting on her make-up, touching herself with a dab of perfume, rubbing moisturizer on her supple, fully intact skin. Put yourself in her busy life, taking care of her husband and kids, moving around in her job as a receptionist, and greeting customers with a smile. A day before, she was fulfilling all the obligations of an active life. Now here she was, immobile, her skin peeling off, the disinfectant smells of the hospital replacing her usual scents, the awareness of the monitors and buzzers replacing her everyday senses. And the disarming assault arose from inside, not from something external like a burn. This mutiny of her vital covering could make her feel as alien to herself as the skin that was being rejected.

"We need to watch you very carefully over the next several days to make sure you don't get an infection or lose too much of your vital fluids," I said. "The skin acts as a barrier to bacteria; therefore we have to take every precaution to protect you until your skin returns in full. As you know, we are made of a high percentage of water. The skin is like a regulator to help make sure the right amount of fluid stays in, and the correct amount goes out. Without skin, you lose the principal way your body maintains a fluid balance." I paused, giving her time to absorb my little speech. "It looks like you've lost most of your skin surface, and it will take some time to get a new one. You need the IV fluids so you don't get dehydrated. And we have to be very careful about infection. Please be patient and hang in."

"I'll be here, Doc," she said.

"I'll need to take a small sample of your skin to send to the pathologist. It will help in confirming your diagnosis."

"Whatever. It's OK," Mary said. "I probably won't feel it too much."

Mary was right; she showed very little discomfort as I anesthetized the irritated skin and used a tiny punch tool to extract a sample. I put it into the biopsy bottle, where the pathologist would take it out later for preparation and examination.

I discussed Mary's situation with Peggy, and thanked her for her time. Next I called Bill Cook and put together a game plan. In Mary's case, we were initially able to stabilize her and improve her condition in the internal medicine unit of our hospital, given the excellent medical care provided in that setting. However, with such a dramatic skin insurrection, after three days of hospitalization I ordered Mary to be transferred to the burn unit, where I felt more comfortable with the highly qualified staff's expertise in dealing with the problems of an acute process like Mary's. An efficient program of fluid administration and its modification according to the needs of the patient being treated can only be carried out with careful, accurate, and current data, most importantly the intake and output of fluid (water from all sources in, urine output). A number of physiologic criteria indicating the efficiency of the fluid therapy must be carefully monitored, including the patient's vital signs (blood pressure, pulse, respiration, temperature) and general condition, the hematocrit, complete blood count, serum electrolytes, and the central venous pressure. The trend of the venous pressure readings from half-hour to half-hour, for example, is usually the first indication of over- or under-replacement of fluid. In addition, topical antibacterial agents are applied to control wound infection. The treatment usually consists of loose gauze dressings saturated with antibacterial ointment applied directly over the denuded skin. And nutritional assessment is crucial to determine metabolic conditions. All of these factors play an integral part in burn injuries, so the burn unit is an excellent place for someone like Mary to be supervised.

I went back, talked with Mary, and explained why we needed to move her. "I agree," she said.

"And I need to get some other folks in to take a peek at you, like an ophthalmologist."

"My eyes have been pretty dry," she offered. "And my mouth."

Mary suffered from toxic epidermal necrolysis, or TEN, which is often a reaction to medication. Most cases sprout 1–3 weeks after starting the drug. If the patient had a similar eruption in the past, the time interval drops to less than 48 hours due to increased sensitization to the offending agent.

Not only is TEN one of the most severe drug reactions, but the condition may progress very rapidly, as it did with Mary. Statistically, one in seven patients lose their entire epidermis in 24 hours. Without this major barrier, the body acts like a party invitation for bad critters. The mouth often dries up, making the oral intake of fluids and food unbearable, which further intensifies the imbalances brought on by loss of skin.

Although TEN is considered exceedingly rare, its frequency may be underestimated because of misdiagnosis of mild and marginal cases. The disease is much more common in adults, but has been described in the medical literature in children. No racial or sexual preponderance has been reported. The disease generally occurs sporadically, but epidemic-like occurrence has been observed with the mass use of sulfonamides for meningitis. The long list of etiologic factors points to an underlying immune mechanism. However, the nature of TEN is still unclear and a matter of speculation.

On Mary's second day of hospitalization, I got the results back of the skin sample I had taken during my initial visit with her. Blisters and dead skin characteristic of TEN were evident, helping to clinch the diagnosis.

The damage of TEN, although not as directly severe as burn trauma, can result in large losses of body fluid through the open wounds brought on by the disease, and large losses of water by surface evaporation. The severity of these changes is directly proportional to the depth and extent of the injuries. The result can be a marked diminution in blood volume, resulting in a fall in cardiac output followed by marked decrease in tissue and organ perfusion. Therefore, in the first 24–48 hours of the disease onslaught, every effort must be made toward replacing fluids lost.

Severe skin injury destroys the protective function of the skin as a barrier to microorganisms. Within a very short time bacteria contaminating the wound surface begin to multiply and proliferate in the area of the wound, and destroyed tissues are an excellent culture medium. The wounds, if untreated, can become the principal site of bacterial infection, with disastrous complications if not controlled. The usual culprits found in the wounds are staphylococci, as well as gram-negative bacteria of which *Pseudomonas* is common. In Mary's case, topical antimicrobial agents such as silver sulfadiazine were used to prevent invasive infection. Iced or cold water applications helped alleviate pain and decrease injury. The wounds were cleansed and dead skin carefully removed and sterile dressings applied. An injection for tetanus prevention was also given;

this is the standard of care for wound patients in which no history (as in Mary's case) of recent tetanus immunization was noted. On occasion, skin excision and grafting is required with severe skin loss, such as with burns, but in my experience with Mary and other TEN patients, localized skin care and biological dressings are often sufficient for recovery.

Systemic signs of TEN can include high fever, high white bloodcell count, elevation of liver enzymes, water and electrolyte imbalance which may proceed to hemodynamic shock, pulmonary edema, and renal failure. Severe involvement of the respiratory and gastrointestinal tracts can result in tracheitis, bronchopneumonia, and esophageal and gastrointestinal hemorrhage. Renal complications, including acute tubular necrosis and glomerulonephritis have also been described.

As a general rule, the mucous membranes are also severely affected. Lips, oral mucosa, conjunctivae, as well as genital and anal mucous membranes show redness and widespread destruction. Fingernails and toenails may be shed, and eyebrows and cilia may slide off, together with the epidermis of the eyelids. In Mary's case, she did suffer from localized erosion inside her mouth, which was readily treated with topical medicines that helped heal and anesthetize the tender sites.

With most skin conditions, such as acne, basal cell cancers, even melanomas, there is a certain sense of time to plan the best course of action. With Mary, this was not the case.

As already noted, the skin has three basic levels – epidermis, dermis, and subcutaneous – from top to bottom. With TEN, the epidermis is the primary level affected. The dermal vessels may swell but no gross damage is noted on microscopic examination. The damage in TEN tends not to be nearly as severe as (third-degree) burn injuries, where a process called "coagulation necrosis" occurs, and total skin loss with scar formation occurs. The recovery from most cases of TEN is more in line with first-degree and superficial second-degree burns, where one may expect healing within a month, although some residual redness may remain for a few weeks.

The damage with TEN is generally so widespread that a patient like Mary is at great risk. Mary had lost her skin, involuntarily, without the atavistic drive that signals a snake to shed, or the normal course of skin loss and regrowth during years of wear and tear. Her loss was in fast motion and unyielding in its destructiveness. We needed to move quickly and aggressively.

TEN's mortality rate is 25-70% depending on the research study quoted. Recovery is slow, and frequent relapses occur. The course and prognosis are highly dependent on quick and adequate treatment. The peak of the disease (by the third day in Mary's case) bears the highest threat, and the fate of the patient often hangs in the balance for one or more weeks. Secondary infection is the most common cause of death. Gastrointestinal hemorrhage and fluid and electrolyte imbalance are other major complications leading to death. Surviving patients heal in 3-4 weeks, but up to 50% have residual and potentially disabling eye lesions, including corneal opacities. Due to improvements in skin and wound care, including faster-acting antibiotics and increasingly effective wound coverings, along with earlier recognition and treatment of TEN, we have improved our ability to treat this condition.

What brings about this terrible eruption?

The etiology of most cases cannot be nailed down, but drugs are the most common culprit. In one study, drugs were implicated in 77% of the cases. Since the average patient with TEN (not Mary) is on 4.4 drugs, it is often problematic to identify the offending drug. Antiepileptic, sulfonamides, ampicillin, and nonsteroidal anti-inflammatories are the most frequent offenders.

I reviewed everything with Peggy, and before I left to go back to my office, I stopped back in on Mary. "I'll see you later today," I said. "When I get done with my office hours, I'll check back and see how you're doing."

"Thanks, Doc," she said. "I'm glad you're on the case. It's not every day that I lose my skin."

I smiled, and nodded in appreciation of her humor under pressure. Later, we found the culprit. The drug she had taken for her ear pain contained sulfa, which was the most likely detonator for the explosion on her skin. After a week in the hospital she improved, and within a month she was up and around. Her eyes appeared to be spared any chronic harm.

When I saw Mary prior to her discharge from the hospital, I gave her a list of all medicines containing sulfa for her avoidance, and told her she was not immune in any way to this disease. In fact, she would be at high risk for recurrence if she took sulfa-containing products again.

I saw Mary again about a month after she left the hospital. Given how dramatic her appearance was in the hospital, she had fared quite well. Most of her skin was back again, like normal, but she still retained a few areas on her skin where she had minimal scarring, such as a spot on her left thigh. After two trips to her eye doctor, she reported she had a little damage to her cornea but would probably have very little, if any, damage to her eyesight.

Although her case was time-consuming, I was glad I had been consulted, and was looking forward to following her progress. It felt good to know there was still a need for a specialist like me to be in a hospital once in a while, and I was glad I could be of service.

Three

NUMBNESS OF THE ARM

"Is there anything else that you can tell me about it? Does it itch? Is it painful?" I asked.

"No, not really," my patient replied. Patrick was a quiet, thin man of 22. He told me he worked in the biology department at a local university, and that he had arrived from Vietnam eight years ago. Since then, he had not traveled outside the United States. He had family in a nearby town and lived off campus in an apartment with a couple of friends.

Patrick's problem was a small growth on his left arm. It was about the size of a nickel, with little pigmentation and ill-defined borders. He told me he'd had the growth for about eight months. I asked him if there were any other trouble spots. He said he also had a bad rash on his left elbow that got itchy on occasion. He also complained of a rash on the left side of his face that had been there for a couple of months. The spot on his left elbow was irregular and irritated. I noticed some slight redness near the growth.

Those features could describe a number of different problems. I was going to recommend a biopsy when he suddenly spoke up and pointed to his arm. "It does feel kind of numb sometimes."

That's when a bell began ringing in my head. I had seen this before, ten years or more ago, on another patient. That patient's growth developed somewhat differently, but the sensation of numbness was the same.

I explained that I would need a biopsy to confirm my diagnosis. Patrick nodded his head. He signed the consent form for the biopsy, and I proceeded to remove a bit of skin. When I was finished, I wrote down what I suspected on the biopsy report, which would be picked up by the lab with the specimen later in the day. I explained to Patrick how to care for the biopsy site, arranged for a follow-up visit, and sent him home.

A couple of days later, the dermatopathologist reported lab results that confirmed my hunch. "First time I've seen this," he said. "Lepromatous leprosy."

The next day I reviewed a copy of the slide containing Patrick's biopsy. Among the skin cells were numerous dark spots: the bacilli of *Mycobacterium leprae*. As required by law, I reported his case to the health department and did the follow-up paperwork.

Mycobacterium leprae was first identified as the cause of leprosy by a Norwegian doctor, Dr G. Armauer Hansen, in 1873. Although leprosy is often thought of as a disease of the tropics, leprosy (or Hansen's disease) has been widespread historically in regions as diverse as Iceland, Scandinavia, North Korea, Japan, and India. An even more common misconception is that leprosy is highly contagious. In fact, most people exposed to the bacterium, which is thought to spread through respiratory droplets, can easily fend it off. But in some people, for some reason, the bacterium takes hold.

Once an infection is established, it can show up in one of three forms. The most severe is lepromatous leprosy, in which the bacterium spreads widely beneath the skin and throughout the body. Another, milder form is tuberculoid leprosy. Its hallmark is severe nerve damage. In particular, the peripheral nerves of the arms and neck can become permanently damaged. The third type, borderline leprosy, occupies the broad and variable zone between lepromatous and tuberculoid leprosy.

The reason for the different forms has to do with how an individual's immune system responds to the bacterium. Immune cells called macrophages normally consume the bacterium, which cannot migrate and releases no toxins. The symptoms of leprosy occur because, in some cases, the macrophages cannot always dispose of *M. leprae*. In tuberculoid leprosy, the immune system manages to isolate the bacteria by walling them off in distinct lesions of infected macrophages. In lepromatous leprosy, the bacterium accumulates and spreads not only in skin cells but also throughout the body. Because the bacterium prefers cooler temperatures, lesions are common in the skin, extremities, and joints.

Left untreated, the disease can form abscesses and ulcers in the skin, spread into the kidneys, and trigger nerve damage and arthritis. In advanced untreated cases, patients can lose fingers and toes. Infected cells can cluster and block blood flow, which can cause tissue to die. Or the clusters can block nerves, causing numbness that puts patients at risk for burns or injuries. Fortunately, most leprosy cases respond very well to treatment. The drug Rifampicin kills 99.98% of leprosy bacilli within a few days.

I teamed up with an infectious disease group to treat Patrick. He was put on antibiotics: Dapsone 100 mg every day along with Rifampicin 600 mg a day. Because Patrick's liver enzymes rose during treatment – a sign of drug toxicity – we decided he needed a different mix of drugs. After consulting with doctors from the US Centers for Disease Control and Prevention we discontinued Rifampicin and added Clofazamine, which fights both bacteria and inflammation.

Patrick proved difficult to treat. He continued to develop adverse reactions to the leprosy. He also missed several appointments and said he couldn't afford the medications. Meanwhile, he developed more reactions, with pain and swelling on the face, particularly on the right cheek. He continued to do poorly and his liver enzymes continued to rise. His total bilirubin, a key liver enzyme, was 6.6 (normal is 0–1.3).

After a few months of treatment, Patrick's bilirubin level went down to 3.2 and continued to fall. But he resisted treatment, and he continued to have brawny, round, inflamed lesions, and swelling and redness on his arms and his face. We consulted a specialist at the National Hansen's Disease Center, who recommended increasing his steroids to bring down the swelling.

Patrick showed a surprising lack of concern about his condition. He was clearly aware of his problem and may have witnessed it as a youngster in Vietnam. The last time I talked with him, the infectious disease specialists to whom I had referred him were treating him. I hoped he was doing better. I felt sure that if he had cooperated more fully at the beginning, he could have enjoyed a much more rapid and effective treatment.

Since 1950, the estimated number of leprosy cases worldwide has fallen from 15 million to perhaps 2 million. In the United States, the disease is rare: there are only about 3,000 cases. Still, leprosy's peculiarities frustrate researchers. Since the 1940s, we've had drugs to treat the disease, but efforts to create a vaccine have failed. One reason is that researchers don't know what conditions *M. leprae* need to survive in the lab. An effective vaccine could eradicate the disease, which remains a significant problem in some regions. India, Myanmar, and Nepal, for example, are home to 70% of leprosy patients.

Given the rarity of leprosy in the United States, it seemed both strange and lucky that I had seen leprosy twice in my eighteen-year career. If I had not seen it the first time, I would not have recognized it the second time.

Four

A MYSTERY

A 32-year-old, Hispanic woman came to see me, accompanied by her parents. She asked about getting a growth taken off her lip. I asked how long it had been there, and she replied "ten years." I performed a history and physical, and noted a raised red bump on her left upper lip, appearing as an irregular hematoma. Graciella was mildly mentally retarded, and the family had moved to Tampa, Florida, from a tough area in New York City about eight years ago. She remembered getting some rocks thrown at her one day by rowdy neighborhood kids. "I think one of them hit my lip," she said, pointing to the raised bump.

As with most events in life, I wondered: why now? "Why after all this time do you want this off?" I asked.

"I don't know," she said. "I'm just tired of looking at it."

I had her sign a consent form after reviewing the procedure with her and her parents. The mother appeared quite anxious, and the parents left the room prior to the procedure.

I numbed up the area, and Graciella seemed to handle everything without much distress. I used a scalpel to open the lesion and explored it with a dissecting scissors. Within a short time, I probed and found a solid object that resembled a small hematoma. Using a pickup, I was ready to pluck it into the biopsy bottle when I noticed something shiny. While Graciella put pressure on the wound, I pressed on the object with my fingertips. The bloody covering slipped off, revealing a tiny copper ball. It was a B-B! I dropped it in the bottle, and it landed with a little "kerplunk."

"I don't think you got hit by a rock ten years ago," I said. "You got shot with a B-B gun."

"A B-B?" she exclaimed. "Oh my God! Momma, Pappa, come here!"

The parents came in; the mother was a bit hysterical when she heard the news.

"That's a first," I said.

Graciella just shook her head in amazement. After ten years, the mystery had been solved.

Five

MELANOMA

"You have a melanoma," I said softly, yet firmly.

Ted Nardone, a big chunk of a man, finally seemed to pay attention to me. He sat on the examining table, his tie at half-mast, looking haggard after a day of work in the world of stocks and bonds. I had taken a skin sample off his back the week before, a small piece from a much larger growth located in the upper center of his five foot eight, 270-pound frame. He had returned for removal of his sutures and a diagnosis.

I placed the suture removal first in his reasons for returning, because I believe he may not have come back to see me otherwise. Nothing in his previous behavior had indicated that he was aware of, or willing to acknowledge, the danger living on his back. A mutual friend of ours, named Chris, had urged Ted to come see me. Chris and Ted had played racquetball together, and Chris had noticed the large black mole on his friend's back. Until recently, Ted had ignored Chris' recommendation to get the growth looked at by an expert.

"I just didn't have time for it," Ted told me. "You know, I'm on the phone from early morning on. And in the evening, I got to get out and socialize to get more clients. And the ladies want my time. You know. It's endless."

"How long has it been on your back?" I asked.

"As far as I know, about two years," he said. "Lately it's been itching a lot."

Ted was a stockbroker, a party animal, a man of expensive tastes and overindulgence, acutely unaware of the limitations of his body. I had to deflate his ego just to get him to fit inside my examining room.

"Am I gonna die, Doc?" Ted asked, a tiny hint of worry in his otherwise haughty voice.

"This is a serious problem," I told him. "You've got to respect the power of this disease, or you can run into major problems. You have a chance of survival if you get this taken care of right away."

Even though I had to send it to the lab for confirmation, I knew it was a melanoma. God knows, Florida seems to be a breeding ground for the malicious beasts.

In diagnosing the malignancy, we use the four basic warning signs of melanoma – ABCD:

- Asymmetry (if a line was drawn through the middle, the two sides don't match);
- Border (irregular in shape, with scalloped or notched edges);
- Color (variety of shades, including mixed red, white, and blue);
- Diameter (larger than ¼ inch, or the size of a pencil eraser).

Ted's tumor showed asymmetry and displayed multiple areas of pigmentation, ranging from slightly pink to dark blue.

As dermatologists, we have years of experience in recognizing patterns. Each dermatologist's mind contains thousands of patterns of lesions observed, and by examining lesions, doing biopsies, and microscopically checking the acquired specimens and confirming the diagnoses, we are able to develop accurate patterns of recognition. Just as a veteran mechanic can listen to the sound of an engine and judge a car's worth, or a practiced florist can put together the right bunch of flowers, the dermatologist is adept at picking out the more ominous lesions among the hundreds of varieties of growths that find a home on our skin.

"Can you take it out now?" Ted asked. "I don't have insurance, and I'd trust you to do it."

"I appreciate your trust," I told him. "But no, I can't."

"Why not?" he asked. "I'll pay you in cash. What about five hundred bucks? I don't have any insurance, and I don't want to go to a hospital or see anybody else."

I wasn't put off by Ted treating his illness like a common commodity that could be bought at a specified price. In eighteen years of practice and 150,000 patients, I've seen all types, with all kinds of understandings of the doctor–patient interaction.

"I know somebody you can see that will work out your financial situation," I told him. "If it were a different type of skin cancer, something less problematic, I would cut it out. But this is too important to not have you seen by the experts. I do general dermatology, but there are others who concentrate primarily on melanomas. That's who you need to see."

I stayed calm, avoiding any hint of being histrionic with Ted. He didn't seem like the type who would be impressed by any theatrics. And I had given up any bullying of patients years ago, knowing that they would arrive at their own pace into the world of realization and acceptance.

I gave Ted copies of all his pathology reports and pertinent office notes and lab data, and gave him the number of a specialist I had in mind, Dr Cruse, who worked at the major teaching hospital in the area – Tampa General. Ted called me back a couple days later, almost begging me to do the surgery myself. I insisted that he go to a specialist and a place where all the proper tests could be performed, including studies of the lymph glands to check for metastases. Finally, he seemed to understand, and I received a preliminary report from Dr Cruse a couple of weeks later.

The biopsy report provides a springboard for further evaluation; however, establishing the diagnosis of melanoma is just the beginning. Classifying the degree of severity is the next step. Extensive physical examination and additional laboratory studies is of vital importance in determining the stage of the melanoma. The stages for a cancer can be compared to the stages of life, considering infancy as stage I, and old age as stage IV. With melanoma, stage I is early and localized and stage IV is advanced and metastasized.

Each stage of melanoma has certain specifications. The early stages (I and II) are classified according to the thickness of the tumor, known as the Breslow's thickness, and by the number of layers of skin invaded by the tumor, known as Clark's level of invasion. Together these two measurements provide a very clear picture of the melanoma and help to recognize its stage.

Breslow's thickness measures in millimeters (1 mm equals 0.04 inch) the distance between the top layer of the epidermis and the deepest point of tumor penetration. Very thin tumors are 0.75 or less, thin tumors 0.76–1.5 mm, intermediate tumors are 1.51–3.99 mm, and thick melanomas 4.0 mm or more. The thinner the melanoma, the better the chance of cure; the Breslow thickness is the key to predicting the progression of the disease.

Let's review. The skin has three major layers: the most superficial is the epidermis, the middle is the dermis, and the lowest is the subcutaneous level. Clark's level I occupies only the epidermis. (The term melanoma in situ refers to a tumor that occupies only the uppermost part of the epidermis.) When a melanoma penetrates to the layer immediately under the epidermis, it is Clark's level II. A Clark's level III melanoma fills a sizable amount of the dermis, level IV penetrates into the deep dermis, and level V invades the subcutaneous fat.

Ted had a Clark's level stage III melanoma. What were his options? And what about his prognosis?

The sooner the cancer is caught and treated, the better the results. The first step in treatment is the removal of the melanoma. Surgical excision, or cutting it out, is the standard method of removing the lesion. Another term for surgical excision is resection, and the borders of the entire area excised are known as the margins. You may have seen the residual scars of those who have had a melanoma removed five or ten years ago, which often are as big as gall bladder scars or other large surgeries. In the past few years, great advances have been made in the surgical technique for melanoma removal, and much less tissue is required for a safe and thorough removal.

With thin melanomas, outpatient procedures under local anesthesia are sufficient. Wound healing generally occurs in 1–2 weeks and scars are minimal. If extensive surgery is required, flaps made from skin that is near the tumor or grafts of skin taken from another part of the body are used to provide cosmetic repair.

Once the melanoma has progressed beyond stage II, as in Ted's case, the key question becomes: Has the tumor spread beyond the original site? If it has spread, the lymph nodes closest to the tumor are the most likely site of metastases.

The quickest way to determine whether the melanoma cells have escaped the primary tumor is for the examining physician to feel the nearby lymph nodes. If the melanoma is on the arm, for example, the nearest nodes are in the armpit. When an enlargement or lump in a lymph node can be recognized by touch, the word used to describe it is palpable. A lymph node that is palpable can be surgically removed in a node biopsy. In Ted's case, I found no swelling in the armpits (axillary nodes) or neck (cervical nodes). The nodes were non-palpable, but it does not mean that no tumor was present.

The newest method, called lymphoscintigraphy, maps the lymph system by using a small amount of a radioactive substance injected at the site of the melanoma. With the help of a scanner, the drainage pattern of the lymph fluid draining from the melanoma to the nodes can be traced. The surgeon can examine the results and remove only the lymph nodes that preferentially receive the fluid, indicating metastases.

Distant metastases may occur in stage IV, which indicates melanoma cells have traveled through the body via the bloodstream, going far from the primary tumor site and perhaps invading distant lymph nodes or internal organs. In that case, the physician may order CT (computerized tomography) scans, in which x-rays of the chest, head, abdomen, and pelvis are taken from multiple angles and then recorded by means of computer technology. Nuclear (radioactive) and MRI (magnetic resonance imaging) scans are also sometimes used.

In stages III and IV disease, additional or adjuvant therapy may follow surgery. Several drugs that act on cancer cells are used in melanoma treatment, either one at a time or in combinations. Chemotherapy with drugs such as Dacarbazine (DTIC), carmustine (BCNU), cisplatin, vincristine, and tamoxifen are utilized.

Immunotherapy advances have been made to help the body's own immune system help itself. Experimental melanoma vaccines are dramatically pursued, and multiple trials are underway for patients in stages III and IV of the disease. The vaccines are given to people who already have the disease to prevent it from getting worse and to promote long-term survival.

Biologic therapy, another type of immunotherapy, makes use of chemicals that occur naturally in the body. The most popular chemical is interferon-alpha, the only systemic drug known to improve five-year survival of stage III patients that has been approved by the US Food and Drug Administration (FDA). Another naturally occurring substance, although experimental, is tumor-necrosis factor. Both of these are produced by white cells (lymphocytes) after contact with viruses of tumor cells and have been shown to kill some tumors including melanomas. In addition, they also have "anti-angiogenic" properties that prevent the formation of new blood vessels that may supply and nourish the tumor. An additional form of experimental immunotherapy for stage IV patients utilizes the naturally-occurring substance interleukin-2, which is a type of substance know as a lymphokine, a chemical normally produced in the body in small quantitics or in lymphocytes specially stimulated to kill malignant cells, including melanoma.

In Tcd's casc, preoperative evaluation included a complete blood count, EKG, chest x-ray, and liver function studies to rule out any abnormalities. A preoperative lymphoscintigraphy was done which showed the presence of tumor in the axillary nodes. The next step was a wide excision of the tumor and bilateral axillary lymph node removals.

In today's medical world of Healthcare Maintenance Organizations (HMOs) and gatekeepers, and restricted access to specialists, many people are scared to venture out into the world of healthcare providers, because of the worry that they may face much frustration, great cost, and deadly delay.

Sam Donaldson, the noted ABC news broadcaster, stated "I know the importance of finding the cancer before it is too late. If a melanoma is treated while it is thin and on the top layer of the skin, the survival rate is close to 100 percent." Donaldson and other high-profile people have written their accounts of personal battles with melanoma, and the public is becoming more aware of the ungenerous and democratic nature of the disease.

I handled Ted's questions, and thought back to the many questions others had asked me over the years.

"Do I have a higher chance of another melanoma?"

Yes, the chances of having another melanoma are greater with a history of melanoma. You need regular check-ups every three months for two years, and then yearly for life. With careful watch, most second melanomas are caught at an early stage and treated by surgical excision.

"Is there a special melanoma diet?"

No, but you'll do better keeping a well-balanced diet with folic acid, vitamins B-6, B-12, C and A; iron, and zinc.

"Is it safe to donate blood?"

In most cases, blood centers will not accept blood from someone who has had cancer.

"Is it contagious?"

No. Melanoma is not transmitted by any type of contact. The increased prevalence of this cancer in families is due to an inherited gene, not contagion.

"Should I avoid the sun?"

The Skin Cancer Foundation recommends that all people avoid the sun to the greatest extent possible, especially during the peak sun hours of 10am to 4pm. Use a sunscreen with an SPF of 15 or greater, and wear a hat and sunglasses.

Those with a fair complexion, blue eyes, and blond hair are the most susceptible to melanoma, along with people who have a history of blistering sunburns during childhood.

"I have a sister that has some dark moles on her skin. Who should she see?"

A dermatologist.

A recent study at the University of Toronto revealed that many family physicians are uncomfortable diagnosing melanoma (78% of 355 family physicians admitted a reluctance). In addition, 60% said they rarely sent patients to a specialist. Many HMOs allow direct access to a dermatologist, so anyone can call and make an appointment.

I have taken care of many people that had these malevolent growths, some only of six months or less in duration, who tragically faced an early demise. What got into somebody like Ted, who waited two years and ignored the tumor until it was almost too late? He seemed filled with an arrogance that death would look in another direction, just for him. I don't think it was vanity; most of the vain types are stereotypical gym-jocks that pose in front of mirrors for hours and question any imperfection. Ted acted like he could simply choose to delay the lingering growth, and also eat too much, party even more, until at the very end he was given a rope to swing back to life by a friend. In reality, he was extremely lucky, although without major lifestyle changes his prognosis for a long, healthy life were limited.

I saw Ted one more time, about ten weeks post-op. No further evidence of tumor or problems related to the surgery were observed. It seemed that some of his ego had deflated out of the hole he had in his back. "I'm glad you got me to the right place," he said. "I didn't realize what a mess I was in."

The real hero is in this case was Chris. He was the one who pushed his friend to get seen. I made the diagnosis, which was important, and Dr Cruse and others also played crucial roles in Ted's care. But if not for Chris, I doubt that Ted would still be alive. In the midst of all the political chaos of medicine, our most important assets still shine – friends and family.

Six

THE EYE OF THE STORM

Candice, a woman in her fifties, had a confession: "I've been having trouble seeing lately, Doc."

"What exactly is going on?" I asked. (Candice was not one to profess ill health unless she really had a problem.)

"First I thought it was my glasses so I cleaned them. Then I took off my glasses and closed one eye at a time. I felt like I was looking through a window. It's like a suspension and it's all moving, and I can't get rid of it."

I did a thorough history and asked about any previous family problems.

"I had an aunt like that. She maybe had a cataract or something. My momma told me about it but I don't remember," Candice said.

I looked her over and quickly got her in to see a colleague who was an ophthalmologist. The doctor called me back with a preliminary report. "Histo spots," she said.

That description set my head into research and reflection mode. I had remembered other patients that had similar complaints to Candice. One I had seen in the emergency room many years before who said she had "Big spider webs all over my eyes that I can't shake." The description of visual occlusion was similar to Candice's.

Both patients had similar backgrounds in one respect – they had spent extensive time in the Ohio and Mississippi River Valleys. And both turned out to have ocular histoplasmosis, a disease caused when airborne spores of the fungus *Histoplasma capsulatum* are inhaled into the lungs, the primary infection site. This microscopic fungus is found throughout the world in river valleys and soil where bird or bat droppings accumulate. It is released into the air when soil is disturbed by, for example, plowing fields, sweeping chicken coops, or digging holes.

Candice admitted to having a parakeet as a child and living in the Ohio farmlands. "I breathed in the fungus and instead of it going just into my lungs, some of it got into my eyes," she said.

Histoplasmosis is generally so mild that it may only produces minor symptoms. If you had histoplasmosis symptoms, you might dismiss them as those from a cold or flu. The body's immune system normally overcomes the infection in a few days without treatment.

However, even mild cases of histoplasmosis can later cause a serious eye disease called ocular histoplasmosis syndrome (OHS) – a leading cause of vision loss in Americans between the ages of 20 and 40. Researchers believe that *Histoplasma capsulatum* (histo) spores spread from the lungs to the eye, lodging in the choroids. The choroids are the layer of blood vessels that provides blood and nutrients to the retina, the light-sensitive layer of tissue that lines the back of the eye. Although scientists have not yet been able to detect any trace of the histo fungus in the eyes of patients with ocular histoplasmosis syndrome, there is good reason to suspect the histo organism as the cause of OHS.

OHS develops when fragile, abnormal blood vessels grow underneath the retina, forming lesions known as choroidal neovascularization (CNV). Left untreated, CNV lesions can turn into scar tissue and replace the normal retinal tissue in the macula. The macula is the central part of the retina that provides the sharp, central vision that allows you to read this page or drive a car. If scar tissue forms, visual messages from the retina to the brain are affected, and vision loss results.

If these abnormal blood vessels leak fluid and blood into the macula, vision is also impaired. When abnormal blood vessels grow toward the center of the macula, they may affect a tiny depression called the fovea. The fovea is the region of the retina with the highest concentration of special retinal nerve cells, called cones. With damage to the fovea and the cones, this straight-ahead vision can be severely impaired and even destroyed. Early treatment of OHS is essential; if the abnormal blood vessels have affected the fovea, controlling the disease will be more difficult. Since OHS rarely affects side, or peripheral vision, the disease does not cause total blindness.

OHS usually has no symptoms in its early stages. The initial OHS infection usually subsides without the need for treatment. Often the only evidence that the inflammation ever occurred is the presence of tiny scars, called "histo spots," which remain at the infection sites. Although histo spots do not generally affect vision, they can result in complications years – sometimes even decades – after the original eye infection. For unknown reasons, histo spots have been associated with the growth of abnormal blood vessels underneath the retina.

OHS symptoms may appear if the abnormal blood vessels cause changes in vision. Straight lines may appear crooked or wavy, or a blind spot may appear in the field of vision; these symptoms signal that OHS has already progressed enough to affect vision.

Candice was one of the unlucky tiny fraction of people infected with the histo fungus that develops OHS. Like most OHS patients, she tested positive for previous exposure to histoplasmosis. The highest incidence of histoplasmosis in the United States occurs in a region often referred to as the "Histo Belt," where up to 90% of the adult population has been infected by histoplasmosis. The region includes all of Arkansas, Kentucky, Missouri, Tennessee, and West Virginia as well as large portions of Alabama, Illinois, Indiana, Iowa, Kansas, Louisiana, Maryland, Mississippi,

Nebraska, Ohio, Oklahoma, Texas, and Virginia. Most cases of histoplasmosis are undiagnosed. Therefore, anyone who has ever lived in an area known to have a high rate of histoplasmosis should consider having their eyes examined for histo spots.

How was Candice diagnosed with OHS?

A careful eye examination (eyes dilated) revealed two conditions:

1. the presence of histo spots, which indicated previous exposure to the histo fungus spores; and
2. swelling of the retina, which signals the growth of new, abnormal blood vessels.

Since fluid, blood, or abnormal blood vessels were present, a diagnostic procedure called fluorescein angiography was done. In this procedure, a dye, injected into Candice's arm, traveled to the blood vessels of the retina. The dye allowed a better view of the CNV lesion, and photographs documented the location and extent to which it has spread. In particular, attention was paid to how close the abnormal blood vessels are to the fovea.

The only proven treatment for OHS is a form of laser surgery called photocoagulation, which is also used in other diseases such as diabetic retinopathy. Clinical trials, sponsored by the National Eye Institute, have shown that photocoagulation can reduce future vision loss from OHS by more than half. The treatment is most effective when the CNV has not grown into the center of the fovea and the entire area of CNV is destroyed.

A small, powerful beam of light was focused on Candice's fragile, abnormal blood vessels, as well as a small amount of the overlying retinal tissue. Although the destruction of retinal tissue during the procedure could itself cause some loss of vision, this was done in the hope of protecting the fovea and preserving the finely-tuned vision it provides.

Like many diseases, OHS cannot be cured. Once someone like Candice contracts it, OHS remains a threat to her sight for her lifetime. And patients with OHS in one eye are likely to develop it in the other. Unfortunate souls such as Candice with OHS who experience one bout of abnormal blood vessel growth may have recurrent CNV, and each recurrence can damage vision and may require additional laser therapy. Therefore, it is crucial to detect and treat OHS as early as possible before it causes significant visual impairment.

After she had been diagnosed, Candice was appreciative of my concern and referral, although much of the damage had already been inflicted. She went on to have several laser treatments and extensive bleeding with a detached retina as a result of one of her procedures. "I was put out of business," she said, reflecting on her previous career as a nurse.

Her vision now is 20/400, which can't be corrected with glasses (20/200 is legally blind). But Candice is considering new laser surgeries that hold promise for vision improvement in the future.

Seven

THE COLOR OF BURN

Frances Pinkham was a mess. Her teeth were rotten and she had a rather foul smell. She had a slightly dazed look, like a lost snowflake in a storm. She came to see me for "spots all over."

I took a closer look. On her sun-exposed areas, cancerous skin was more prominent than normal skin.

"I just got insurance. Ain't had it in more than ten years. Reckoned I better get in and see if a skin doctor could help me."

As we talked, the problem behind her skin cancers became clearer. She wore sunglasses. When she removed them, she showed signs of nystagmus – irregular rapid movement of the eyes back and forth – and strabismus – muscle imbalance of the eyes ("crossed eyes" or "lazy eye"). The sunglasses reflected her sensitivity to bright light and glare. "I can't see too good," she said.

Frances had albinism. Her chief diagnosis was oculocutaneous albinism, which carries a number of signs and symptoms, including extremely poor visual acuity (most victims are legally blind).

Frances had developed a huge basal cell cancer on her right temple. I removed a piece for pathological inspection. I asked her if she knew much about her albinism. "Somebody once told me something about it, but I can't remember much."

So, what is albinism?

The word "albinism" refers to a group of inherited conditions. People with albinism have little or no pigment in their eyes, skin, or hair; they have inherited albinism genes (from both parents) that do not make the usual amounts of a pigment called melanin. The exception is one type of ocular albinism, which is passed on from mothers to their sons.

Albinism was noted in the earliest medical literature. Several Greek and Roman authors (including Plinius Secundus the Elder and Aulus Gellius) described albinism in humans. Tyrosinase deficiency in animals was first demonstrated in 1904, and the first accurate scientific paper written about albinism was by Sir Archibald Garrod in 1908.

In the US and in the UK, one person in 17,000 has some type of albinism. Albinism affects people from all races. Most children with albinism are born to parents who have normal hair and eye color for their ethnic backgrounds. Often people do not recognize that they have albinism.

What do people with albinism look like?

Most people with albinism look like Frances, with very light skin and hair. In less pigmented types of oculocutaneous albinism (the type of albinism that affects both the skin and the eyes), hair and skin are cream-colored. In types with slight pigmentation, hair appears more yellow or red-tinged. People with ocular albinism (albinism that only affects the eyes) usually have normal or only slightly lighter than normal physical appearance.

A common myth is that people with albinism have red eyes. Different types of albinism exist, and the amount of pigment in the eyes varies. Although some individuals with albinism have reddish or violet eyes, most, like Frances, have blue eyes, but others may have hazel or brown eyes.

The striking appearance of albinism has fascinated humankind for centuries, drawing reactions ranging from veneration to alienation. In some Asian societies dating back to ancient times, and in Europe during the Middle Ages and the Renaissance, fair skin was considered very attractive, a sign of wealth and high social status. Tanned skin meant that one was obligated to work in the fields for one's livelihood. Similarly, the powdered white wig worn by American colonial era illuminati reflected the wearer's ability to afford luxury items and be identified as one of the educated elite.

Nevertheless, in 19th-century America, albinism was considered such a bizarre trait that people with this condition were exhibited in circus sideshows. Furthermore, with the advent of the camera, these individuals were featured on postcards, which were widely distributed and collected from the 1870s to the 1890s. Photo studios such as those of Charles Eisenmann, Obermuller & Son, and Matthew Brady specialized in taking pictures of what were regarded as human oddities.

Even today, a plethora of misconceptions about albinism persists. Bizarre characters (usually villains) labeled "albinos" with snow-white skin and hair, blood-red eyes, and supernatural powers plague the entertainment industry. Many people with albinism have been institutionalized and/or stripped of educational and vocational opportunities due to a misguided belief that the visual impairment accompanying the condition prevents one from being able to adequately function in and contribute to society. Some members of the medical profession have even been known to recommend abortions to mothers carrying babies with albinism because it was thought that their children would die at an early age and would fail to lead productive lives.

Many Native American and South Pacific tribes believed that human beings and animals with albinism were messengers from divine entities. Some saw them as good omens and treated them with utmost respect. Others viewed their presence as a manifestation of wrongdoings within the tribe. In Africa, life has always been particularly difficult for people with albinism. Widespread poverty and ignorance about the condition deprives these individuals of much-needed protection from the burning sun. As a result, many die prematurely from skin cancer. Even if they do manage to avoid the strong sunlight, it often means a life of virtual solitary confinement and prohibition from participating in the daily activities of their kinship group.

I have had other patients with this disease. One was a man named Moses Akhu, who had grown up in South Africa. "I'm new to this country," Moses said. "Things were not good where I came from. Because of my skin people there thought I was evil." We had discussed his history and he revealed he had been kept out of school and almost totally ostracized in his community because of his condition. And, like Frances, he was afflicted with skin cancers.

People with albinism are still at risk of isolation, because the condition remains often misunderstood. Social stigmatization can occur, especially within communities of color, where the race or paternity of a person with albinism may be questioned. Families and schools must make an effort not to exclude children with albinism from group activities.

In the western world, people with albinism live normal life spans and have the same types of general medical problems as the rest of the population. If they use appropriate skin protection, such as sunscreen lotions rated factor 20 or higher, and wear opaque clothing, people with albinism can enjoy outdoor activities even in summer. However, those who do not use skin protection may develop life-threatening skin cancers.

People with albinism have average vision of 20/200, may be either far-sighted or near-sighted, and often have astigmatism. They are sensitive to glare, but people with albinism do not prefer to be in the dark, and need light to see just like anyone else. Visual impairment in albinism results from abnormal development of the retina and abnormal patterns of nerve connections between the eye and the brain. The retina, the surface inside the eye that receives light, does not develop normally before birth and in infancy. The nerve signals from the retina to the brain do not follow the usual nerve routes. The iris, the colored area in the center of the eye, lacks sufficient pigment to screen out stray light coming into the eye. (Light normally enters the eye only through the pupil, the dark opening in the center of the iris, but in albinism light can pass through the iris as well.) It is the presence of these eye problems that defines the diagnosis of albinism. The main test for albinism is simply an eye exam.

For the most part, treatment of eye conditions in albinism consists of visual rehabilitation. Surgery to correct strabismus may improve the appearance of the eyes. However, since surgery will not correct the misrouting of nerves from the eyes to the brain, it will not provide fine binocular vision. In the case of esotropia or "crossed eyes," surgery may help vision by expanding the visual field (the area that the eyes can see while looking at one point). Sunglasses or tinted contact lenses help outdoors. Indoors it is important to place lights for reading or close work over a shoulder rather than in front.

Later I did a more aggressive surgery on Frances and removed the remainder of her facial skin cancer. Over the following weeks I did more gardening of her cancer-ridden fields of skin. I checked over the surgical sites and there were no signs of infection. I reviewed sun protection and care of the surgical sites with her.

Due to her condition, it was difficult for Frances to see the results of her surgeries, but I told her it looked a whole lot better. "That's what people say," she said. "It feels better, too." She seemed pleased, a smile crossing the pink sky of her face.

Eight

A HAIRY TALE

I had a six-year-old African-American girl in front of me named Alisia, with patches of hair loss that looked like a bad mower had gone over the bumpy lawn of her hair.

"How long has it been?" I asked.

"About six months," her mother answered.

The differential diagnoses for hair loss swam through my mind.

First, as with all consultations, I had to focus on the age of the patient, and the location and distribution of the problem.

Changes in the hair can be a huge trickster. That's why the age and condition of the patient is so important. For example, when a woman is pregnant, more of her hairs will be growing. After a woman delivers her baby, many hairs enter the resting phase of the hair cycle. Within 2–3 months, some women will notice large amounts of hair coming out in their brushes and combs. This can last 1–6 months, but resolves completely in most cases. I've seen woman, chasing remedies that are unnecessary, pouring more money down the drain than the hair that is lost.

I had seen all kinds of hair loss before, but Alisia's particular pattern threw me off. I began to ask questions that could point to a diagnosis.

"What kind of treatments has she had?"

Alisia was an involuntary star of the stage, propped up on the examining table, with a shy, courteous smile. "She got some of this," Alisia's mother said, and offered me a bottle.

I looked it over. Alisia had been given an anti-fungal shampoo, which is a common gut-reaction move on the part of most pediatricians. Fungus infection (Ringworm) of the scalp, a contagious disease that has nothing to do with worms, can be the culprit in hair loss. Scalp infections are endemic in many children like Alisia and so I examined her scalp in detail. However, I did not note anything resembling the disease, including the small patches of scaling that could spread and result in broken hair, redness, swelling, and even oozing. In severe cases, children can get huge lymph nodes and have to be admitted into the hospital for intravenous antibiotics.

"Any recent illnesses or surgery?" I asked.

"Nope."

Severe illnesses or infections and high fever may cause hairs to enter the resting phase. Four weeks to three months after a high fever, severe illness or infection, a person may be shocked to see a lot of hair falling out. This shedding also usually corrects itself, but people who have a severe chronic illness may shed hair indefinitely.

I checked Alisia's throat and neck. Both an over-active thyroid and an under-active thyroid can cause hair loss. Hair loss associated with thyroid disease can be reversed with proper treatment.

Anyone who has a major operation may notice increased hair shedding within one to three months afterwards, but the condition usually reverses itself within a few months.

"What about her diet?"

"I've tried to get her to eat better, you know."

Some people who go on crash diets that are low in protein, or who have severely abnormal eating habits, may develop protein malnutrition. The body will save protein by shifting growing hairs into the resting phase. Massive hair shedding can occur two to three months later. Hair can then be pulled out by the roots fairly easily. This condition can be reversed and prevented by eating the proper amount of protein and, when dieting, maintaining adequate protein intake.

Iron deficiency occasionally produces hair loss. Some people don't have enough iron in their diets or may not fully absorb iron; women who have heavy menstrual periods may develop iron deficiency. Low iron can be detected by laboratory tests and can be corrected by taking iron pills. High doses of vitamin A may also cause hair shedding.

"Any medication?"

Some prescription drugs may cause temporary hair shedding. Examples include some of the medicines used for the following: gout, arthritis, depression, heart problems, high blood pressure, or stroke.

Some cancer treatments will cause hair cells to stop dividing. Hairs become thin and break off as they exit the scalp. This occurs 1–3 weeks after the treatment and patients can lose up to 90% of their scalp hair. The hair will regrow after treatment ends, but patients may want to get wigs before treatment.

Women who lose hair while taking birth control pills usually have an inherited tendency for hair thinning. If hair thinning occurs, a woman can consult her gynecologist about switching to another birth control pill. When a women stops using oral contraceptives, she may notice that her hair begins shedding two or three months later. This may continue for six months by which time it usually stops, similar to hair loss after the birth of a child.

I have seen people lose their hair in all kinds of ways. Hair loss and hair deformities are part of several, mostly exotic, syndromes. Alopecia areata is quite common, however, and is characterized by single or multiple patches of well-demarcated hair loss. Alopecia totalis occurs when total or near-total scalp alopecia is present, and alopecia universalis results in generalized loss of all body hair. Most alopecia occurs in the third to fifth decades of life. Some men who lose most of their scalp hair (and some women) may opt to shave it off completely until their hair rebounds and grows again.

Hair is an odd phenomenon.

Do you know you once had hair all over your face? Only your palms and soles of your feet were not hairy. But you will not see your hairy self in the family photo album: perhaps in the future, but not now. The hair I am referring to is lanugo, the silky and fine hair that starts around the mouth and eyebrows about five months after you've been conceived and are floating around in the womb. And then what happens? All your hair falls off a month before your birth.

How do you know which hair color you will have?

There are really only two colors – a brown and a red. Your genes may decide only to use the red, which gives you red hair. If your hair is extremely brown we call it black. Perhaps the genes decide to use the brown very lightly – you'll have blond hair. But what happens to your hair color as you get older? If you start out red or black, you'll most likely stay red or black. Brown hair will generally get darker, and if you start out blond you can stay blond or go to any shade of brown.

And when you do get hair, which hair color has the most?

Blonds apparently have more fun, and they also have more hair: around 140,000 of them. People with black or brown hair have 110,000, and red hair 90,000. Your hair grows about six inches a year, though a bit faster if you're male. All hair grows a little faster in the summertime (all that rain and sunshine). The hair on your eyebrows and eyelashes never reaches an inch long before falling out. In the race against the toenails, the hair wins out. Fingernails only grow about an inch a year and toenails only about ¾ of an inch.

Our hair falls out at a rate of about 80–100 per day, last time I counted. About 90% of your hair is now growing and about 10% is in a resting stage – just chillin' for about 100 days before it falls out.

If left uncut hair will usually grow to a maximum of 2–3 feet. In 1780 a head of hair measuring 12 feet in length and dressed in a style known as the Plica Polonica (braided hair closely matted together) was sent to Dresden after adorning the head of a Polish peasant woman for 52 years. The braid of hair was 11.9 inches in circumference. Swami Pandarasannadhi, the leader of the Tirudaduturai monastery, Tanjore district, Madras, India, was reported in 1949 to have hair 26 feet in length, but no photographic or scientific evidence has ever been supplied in order to support this claim. In March 1989 a record length of 21 feet was claimed for the hair of 74-year-old Mata Jagdamba, a Yogin living in Ujjain, North India.

We once lived in the days of big hair.

In the 1770s big hair was in vogue. The women used a mixture of horsehair, their own hair, and greased wool, stuck in place with water and flour, to make a creation three feet tall or higher. Wig styles included names such as Elephant, Prudence Puff, Rhinoceros, Cauliflower, Hedgehog, Rose Bag, She-dragon, and Staircase. To add to the display, women put in jewelry, lace, vases containing live flowers, ship models, fruit, stuffed birds, and other assorted goodies. Women riding in carriages had to bend down to keep their hair in one place and doorways had to be raised. And since it took most of the day to fix these up, women sometimes would wait a month or more afterward to wash and comb. Bugs infested the hairdos and women would use long sticks and pins to scratch and make openings in the hair for the critters to escape to less hairy habitats.

In the 17th century the wig was a sign of social status. People in higher paying professions wore the bigger hairpieces and were known as "big wigs." Some goofy guys, circa 1773, wore wigs that stood a foot and a half above their heads and placed a tiny hat on top. The wigs were called Macaroni wigs, and Yankee Doodle imitated these men when he "Stuck a feather in his cap and called it Macaroni". And of course, where there was a profit to be made, there were thieves. The wig stealers of 18th-century London walked through crowds toting hefty baskets on their shoulders. Little boys would pop out of the baskets and steal the wigs off unsuspecting folks and then disappear back inside their hideaways.

How about blue hair like Marge Simpson?

Queen Nefretiri of Ancient Egypt wore a bright blue wig, while the Ancient Greeks of Athens dyed their hair blue, and then dusted it with red, gold, or white powder. The men from Saxon and Gaul tribes in the Dark Ages dyed their mustaches blue to frighten their enemies. What about the little old ladies whose blue hair you see just over the steering wheel of their car? Because white hair tends to develop a yellow tint, hairdressers sometimes apply a light blue color to get rid of the yellow; over several treatments, the hair gets more and more blue. But unless you are a Kerry blue terrier, which grows a dark blue-gray fur, you won't have naturally blue hair.

Want to curl up and dye?

Join the California surfers who use a mixture of hair bleach and Bisquick to make their curls a surf-foam white.

Or what about adding on more hair?

Llama fur implant on your chest, black bear on the central part of your back – let's spice up those tattoos! What about the fond memory of your childhood home on your abdomen, complete with a luxuriant green grass? Live on the edge! (Not the real thing, of course, but a genetic hybrid cooked up in the lab.)

Hairy urban legends abound, and at one time or another I have been asked about most them.

"If I shave or cut my hair will it grow back thicker?"

The base of your hair in your scalp doesn't know what's happening to the rest of it. It will grow back the same way no matter if you shave, cut, or burn it off.

"If I rub my head will the hair grow in that spot?"

No way. Rub-a-dub-dub, no more hair in the tub. Rubbing or massage will not increase circulation significantly; the scalp already has more blood in it than most body parts.

"If I eat bread crusts my hair will turn curly?"

Sorry. Even if you twirl your hair while eating the bread, it ain't happening.

"If you are a woman and go out in public in Carrizozo, New Mexico, without shaving your legs (and your face, if necessary), is it illegal?"

Last time I checked, that's true.

Now, back to Alisia. What was the one question I did not ask? It was a question that would solve the puzzle, and the answer was something that I have seldom heard voluntarily given on the part of the patient.

I leaned down and sat next to Alisia. (It is always better to be at eye level, especially if discussing a potentially uncomfortable subject. All experienced waiters know they get bigger tips when they bend down and go eye level with their patrons.)

"Do you ever pull your hair?" I asked.

She looked up at me, then put her head down again and nodded.

Hair pulling, also called Trichotillomania, occurs when children, and sometimes adults, twist or pull their hair, brows or lashes until they come out. In children especially, this is often just a bad habit that gets better when the harmful effects of that habit are explained. Sometimes hair pulling can be a coping response to unpleasant stresses and occasionally is a sign of a serious problem needing the help of a mental health professional.

Trichotillomania falls into the category of manipulative dermatoses. The existence of this category of disease allows the practitioner to dig a little deeper into the psychological triggering of cutaneous disease. Each pulled hair releases emotional tension. And each hair is fractured at different distances from the scalp that accounts for the ragged alopecia.

I looked up at Alisia's mother. "Has she gone through much stress lately?"

She looked at me and then at Alisia. "Oh yeah. You bet. We moved out of the house about a year ago. Had to. Her Daddy and I weren't getting along."

"I think that might have something to do with it. What do you think, Alisia?" I asked. Again she nodded her head.

"Show me what you do when you pull on your hair," I said. "But don't really yank it out."

She looked up at me as she found a clump of remaining hair, twisted it around her fingers, and pulled skyward. "OK," I said. "Thanks."

Alisia put her hand back on her lap.

"It's been tough on you, hasn't it?" I said.

"Yes," she said, soft as a hair falling on a pillow.

"You think the hair you are losing might be from pulling on it?" I asked.

"Maybe," she said. "I can feel it come off when I do that."

"I think so, too," I said. "And you are worrying your mom when you lose all that hair. Maybe when you feel stressed or angry you can talk to her about it, OK? And leave your hair alone. You are way too pretty to not have a full head of hair."

She smiled and nodded again. "OK."

About six weeks later I saw Alisia and her mother again. The hair had started to return, and she had a more lively and upbeat glow.

I looked at my own hair in the mirror. I am one of the only men I know in my forties whose hair has not receded too far from its original shoreline. In the 1960s I tried to pull my hair down as far as I could to imitate the Beatles. At one time I had an "Afro" and used a pick. But for the last 15 years or so I have kept my hair reasonable and professional. During Hallowe'en, however, I like to wear a Rasta-style wig and imagine what it is like to have that much hair. But then I get hot and take it off.

Nine

LITTLE BUBBLES

"Dr Norman, it's Roger C." My nurse handed me Roger's chart. I picked up the phone.

59-year-old Roger, a patient of mine for many years, sounded distressed. "Doc, I broke out over the left side of my face with these little bubbles. Can I get in to see you? I know you can figure this out."

I was in between patients on a busy afternoon and checked my watch. Roger's clinical image was forming in my mind. However, it was still hazy and greatly in need of refinement; I was hesitant to jump to any conclusions before seeing him and checking in greater detail.

"OK, can you get in here within the next hour?"

"I'm in my car," he said. "See you soon."

I laughed. Typical Roger – tough, dynamic, and always on the move.

I kept seeing my patients. Roger arrived, signed in, and was later put into a consulting room. I walked in, shook his hand, and took a look. He had small mountains of blisters that covered much of his left upper face – forehead, temple, nose, and the area around his eye. The outbreak stopped along the midline of the face as if an invisible barrier existed to block its encroach to the other half. I made a preliminary diagnosis in my mind before I sat down, but it was still appropriate to do a thorough history; the discipline of medicine requires that I ask the important questions first.

"How long have you had this, Roger?" I asked.

"Too long," he said, trying to maintain his composure. His face, however, was not reflective of a happy turn of events. "I just came back from a business trip to San Francisco. I started to feel kind of itchy and had some pain over the last few days. This morning I had burning pain and tingling and my face was really sensitive. But I couldn't see any rash or anything. Yesterday I started getting this rash and then the bubbles and my eyes got red."

"I see," I replied as I looked him over.

"Is this some kind of sexually transmitted disease? Am I gonna die?"

"No," I said. "It looks like shingles. Herpes zoster is the medical name for shingles. Not like the other kind of herpes. This is chickenpox the second time around."

"Is it contagious?"

"The virus that causes zoster can only be passed on to others who have not had chickenpox and then they will develop chickenpox, not zoster," I said. "Zoster is much less contagious than chickenpox. And you can only transmit the virus if your blisters are broken."

"Very frustrating. Worst of all I could give it to my 16-year-old daughter – somehow she escaped getting it when she was younger."

Anyone who's had chickenpox (varicella-zoster virus) can develop herpes zoster. The reactivation of the chickenpox virus occurs when the body's immunity to the virus breaks down. Normal aging, physical or emotional stress, fatigue, poor nutrition, certain medications, chemotherapy, radiation therapy, or other factors may allow the dormant pox virus to come out of hiding in nerve root cells of the body. The virus travels along nerve fibers and settles in fairly isolated areas of skin on one side of the body.

The majority of people who develop zoster are otherwise healthy. However, it is possible for the disease to be reflective of other medical problems including AIDS, and chest x-ray or blood studies sometimes are required to rule out other problems.

"Have you had this before?"

"No," he said, "And I hope I never get it again."

"I don't blame you," I said. "I would think it feels horrible."

"It does."

Without knowing it, I was working under the extended diagnostic shadow cast by Dr von Bokay who, in 1888, observed how susceptible children acquired chickenpox after coming in contact with zoster-infected individuals. I have had many similar reports from nursing homes I work in, where nurses have reported that several of the young workers "come down with chickenpox" after caring for patients with zoster.

So, what is herpes zoster?

Herpes zoster, also known as "shingles" or "zoster," is brought on by a single member of the herpes virus family, varicella-zoster virus (VZV). Varicella or chickenpox has the same etiological agent. At some time during their lives, about 20% of people who have had chickenpox will get zoster. Most people will get zoster only once.

The incidence of zoster is 1.5 to 3.0 cases per 1,000 persons per year; after the age of 75 it is 10 cases per 1,000 persons per year. The new childhood vaccine to prevent chickenpox will decrease the number of future cases of zoster.

The first symptom of zoster is the unilateral rash that soon turns into groups of blisters that look a lot like chickenpox. The infected area of the body usually has severe pain, itching, redness, and numbness. Within a few days of their appearance on the skin, the vesicles break open and form scabs.

Herpes zoster is a great masquerader. During training I admitted a woman to the hospital with chest pain. It turned out four days later, after a batch of uninformative tests, that the pain was the prodromal phase of herpes zoster. I was relieved for her that it wasn't cardiac damage and also humbled by the advent of a tricky disease.

The zoster blisters start out clear but then pus or dark blood collects in the blisters before they crust over (scab). After two or three weeks the blisters disappear but the pain may last longer. In unusual circumstances it is possible to have pain without blisters, or blisters without pain.

Approximately 80–90% of cases resolve spontaneously over 6 months. Persistent segmental pain (post-herpetic neuralgia) occurs in approximately 8% at 30 days and 4.5% at 60 days.

"I want you to know that we will treat this and I will follow you along as you recover," I said. "We're in this together and I'm sure you'll do fine once all this passes."

"Thanks, Doc," he said. "I'm glad you're on my side."

"So was it a tough trip?"

"My business meeting turned out OK but I'm not sure it was worth all this."

"I want you to get an ophthalmology consult," I told him. "Anytime you have this around the eye there's a chance it can be in the eye and I don't want to take any chances with your vision."

Zoster is most common on the trunk and buttocks. The blisters can appear on the arms or legs if nerves in these areas are involved. But it can also appear on the face, as with Roger. Great care is needed if the blisters involve the eye, which are connected to nerves that may be infected with the herpes zoster virus and result in permanent damage.

Blisters on the tip of the nose signal possible eye involvement. Ramsay Hunt syndrome type I – a common complication of shingles – is also known as herpes zoster oticus. The syndrome, which is caused by the spread of the varicella-zoster virus to facial nerves, is characterized by intense ear pain, a rash around the ear, mouth, face, neck, and scalp, and paralysis of facial nerves. Other symptoms may include hearing loss, vertigo (abnormal sensation of movement), and tinnitus (abnormal sounds). Taste loss in the tongue and dry mouth and eyes may also occur.

The usual shingles rash can spread from an involved area of the forehead or cheek to the upper or lower eyelids. Shingles may cause redness of the conjunctiva (the mucous membrane covering the white of the eye). It can also cause small scratches or scarring of the cornea. The scratches on the cornea may increase the risk of bacterial infection in the eye. Shingles may also cause inflammation inside the eye, known as iritis or uveitis and can also affect the optic nerve or the retina.

"What about treatment?" Roger asked.

"Zoster usually clears on its own in a month and seldom recurs. I'm going to give you some pain relievers; also use cool compresses which help to dry the blisters. I'm giving you a topical anesthetic to apply to painful areas. I'm putting you on oral anti-viral drugs that can be prescribed to decrease the duration of skin lesions. These drugs rarely cause headache, stomach upset or lightheadedness. We have stronger medicines but I want to keep those in reserve if and when we need them. I'm also recommending lubricating eye drops until you can get to the ophthalmologist."

I hoped Roger would not suffer from the residual pain of post-herpetic neuralgia after his skin had healed. In severe cases of zoster, the rash can leave permanent scars, long-term pain, numbness, and skin discoloration. The neuralgia can last for months or even years and is more common in older people.

A secondary bacterial infection of the blisters can occur and result in delayed healing. If pain and redness increase or reappear, antibiotic treatment may be needed. Another complication of zoster (or chickenpox), although rare, is the spread of zoster all over the body or to internal organs. Both of these complications tend to occur in those with a weakened immunity.

Roger had residual pain for about two weeks after the rash disappeared. When I saw him again his facial rash had cleared and he was in better spirits. However, the infection did leave him with residual corneal scarring and he required long-term ophthalmologic treatment to avoid visual damage.

"I didn't know those little bubbles could be such a problem," he said. "But I'm glad I saw you when I did. Thanks."

"Glad to help," I said. "You're busy enough without having to worry about those bubbles."

He laughed with the confidence of having fought another battle in life. Although it left its scars, it didn't bring him down for too long.

Ten

A LIFE ON THE SKIN

Adam
Had 'em.
(*On the Antiquity of Microbes*, Anon;
reputed to be the shortest poem in the English language)

I inspected our front yard sago palm on a clear fall day, and noted a thin coating that looked like frost, except this was Tampa, Florida and the temperature was 80 degrees. The sparkling sun revealed an infestation of Asian cycad scale (*Aulacaspis yasumatsui*), a blight that sucks the life out of King and Queen sago palm trees. The microscopically tiny white insect, about 3,000 per square inch, has a tough armor coating and multiplies faster than a duck crossing a superhighway with its tail on fire. In a few months, a 15-foot Queen sago with a spread of over 20 feet will be covered, stems and leaves, with a scale of the nasty beasts. The critters are difficult to eradicate. Even though they don't fly with wings, they can become airborne and spread. When there is a strong wind, the immature form of the insect will land on a sago up to half a mile away. If left uncontrolled, they will eventually kill the plant. I searched the Internet and found a few helpful tips to help my friend from certain demise.

But what minutiae inhabit us?

Luckily, except for a few exceptions, we can fight the critters that float through the air and land on our skin. But as a dermatologist, I have treated tens of thousands of my fellow *Homo sapiens* who have had skin diseases brought on by fungal, bacterial and viral invaders.

Here was my patient Theresa, a feisty 26-year-old character who worked at one of the local exotic dance clubs (a major industry in the West coast of Florida, along with the business of churches and beach resorts and other jobs tied in with skin and salvation). I had treated a friend of hers for another problem with success. On her friend's recommendation Theresa showed up on my office doorstep one day, desperate to get rid of a "bad rash." She wanted to get back to work and the big bucks. And her boss told her to get it taken care of as soon as possible.

"This, like, rash shows up under the lights at work," she told me and my medical student – an eager young woman trainee named Jackie. Theresa lifted her blouse to show how the rash covered her upper back. "I asked some of the other dancers to give me some ideas to get rid of it. But, like, it's dirty in that place and I probably caught it there." No matter what they had dreamed up to remedy the situation, the rash had not gone away.

After I shut the door and turned off the lights, I showed Jackie how the fungus on Theresa's back, *Tinea versicolor*, fluoresced under my handheld diagnostic black light. I made sure Jackie touched the rash. One of my goals as a clinical instructor is to guide a student who is dermatologically visually illiterate to see the important patterns of the more common skin diseases. This also requires feeling for the subtle changes that occur on the skin surface. Sometimes I must hold the hands of timid students as they feel the disease along with taking a visual snapshot, so the hand–eye coordination etches a complete picture in the student's mind. Along with the story from the patient, a more accessible grasp of many diseases is afforded in dermatology than in any other diagnostic discipline.

"That's the same thing," Theresa exclaimed as she looked at herself.

I prescribed her a combination of treatments – pills, cream, and shampoo – for as rapid a relief as possible. "Thanks so much," she said.

"Be patient," I said. "It takes time for it to go away."

We are simply one of over two million species of animals and plants. And, like our fellow mortal inhabitants, we are at the mercy of the tiny virus, bacterium, or yeast. Our skin accounts for approximately 16% of our total body weight and varies in thickness from 1 mm on the eyelids to 3 mm between the shoulder blades and on the palms and soles. People who habitually go barefoot may have soles 1 cm thick. Each of us has about as many bacteria and yeasts on the surface of his or her skin as there are people on earth. The life that lives upon us not only puts our lives in perspective but also allows us a peek at a world within the worlds of our integument, perhaps strange to fathom, yet amazing.

Excuse the pun, but it is all a question of scale. Fleas have parasites. Bacteria can parasitize the parasites of fleas. Viruses can parasitize the same bacteria. As Jonathan Swift put it:

So, nat'ralists observe, a Flea
Hath smaller Fleas that on him prey,
And these have sammler yet to bite 'em,
And so proceed *ad infinitum*. (*On Poetry*, 1733)

What if the yeast *T. versicolor* that is so prodigious in humid climates such as Florida, where as many as 40% of us are known to be infected at any one time, went unchecked like the Asian cycad scale?

Yeasts and fungi are inhabitants of the human skin. A yeast is a single-celled fungus which reproduces by budding. The daughter cell grows out from the parent and eventually breaks free. *Pityrosporum*, which belongs to the family *Cryptococcaceae*, is the most common yeast on our skins. The genus *Pitrosporum ovale* are oval spheres about 2 microns wide and 4 microns long which flourish on our hair and fatty parts of our skin. The scalp and around the nose are prime areas where the *Pitrosporum ovale* popluation can total half a million per square cm. *Pityrosporum orbiculare* – a round yeast of about 2 microns – can bring on problems when it turns into another form. Filaments called *hyphae* expand into a spreading mycelium or root-like growth of fungus.

I have often seen patients with yeast infections following the chronic use of steroid creams and ointments. Steroids are helpful to calm the inflammation of diseases such as eczema, but they also can suppress the body's natural immune defenses, which sets up yeast for a sumptuous feast.

Or what if *Demodex folliculorum* staged a revolution?

What do you think of when you think of mites? The disease-filled Middle Ages? *Demodex* is as jovial and well-adjusted, if I may be anthropomorphic: on clean hair as on dirty and craves blue blood as much as red. The parasites of the human body, in fact, have shown no respect for social order or class as they have evolved with us through the millennia.

Demodex mites are part of normal human fauna. The mites are in the order *Arachnida*, along with mites, ticks, spiders, and scorpions. *Demodex* mites are common commensals of the pilosebaceous unit in mammals. However, there is no consensus to what degree the mites are causative of the skin pathology and how they might contribute to disease.

Demodex, each a third of a millimeter long, is our constant miniature companion throughout life. Although the effect of their presence is still in dispute, as many as 25 mites have been found hanging on to one human eyelash root, which questions their benignity. Each of their individual movements, due to their size, is below the threshold to sensory perception.

As Michael Andrew writes of *Demodex* in his 1976 book *The Life That Lives on Man*:

Nothing amongst all the unsuspected secrets of one's skin is more astonishing than the thought that the roots of one's eyelashes are colonized by mites. Few people can confront with equanimity the idea that worm-like creatures which have been likened to eight-legged crocodiles squirm out their diminutive lives in warm oily lairs in our hair follicles.

Demodex folliculorum usually involves the face and *Demodex brevis* commonly infests the chest and back. Rosacea, a multiphasic disease, is associated with flushing, erythrosis, papulopustular rosacea and phymas; each phase is likely to have its own treatment. *Demodex* is an important factor in the inflammatory reaction. *Helicobacter pylori* has also been associated with rosacea.

In immunocompromised hosts *Demodex* may overpopulate and bring on dermatitis. The related follicle mite in dogs (it appears identical but is unable to live on man) is responsible for mange. *Demodex* mites are implicated in demdectic alopecia or "human mange."

> Pull down thy vanity, it is not man
> Made courage, or made order, or made grace,
>   Pull down thy vanity, I say pull down.
> Learn of the green world what can be thy place
> In scaled invention or true artistry,
> Pull down thy vanity […]
> The green casque has outdone your elegance.
> (Ezra Pound, *Canto 81*, 1948)

What else of our normal flora?

The skin is sterile at birth but only remains so briefly. Examining the umbilicus for *Staphylococcus aureus* shows 25% colonization in the first day of life with a steady increase from then on. We have two types of normal skin flora – transient and resident. Resident flora are capable of multiplication and survival and are found as the dominant component in most skin areas. Resident populations on our skins and cilia (sweeping bristles) in our air passages generally protect us from the incursions of foreign organisms.

Resident flora include *propionibacterium acnes* – a prototype anaerobic diptheroid, found in large numbers with the sebaceous follicles of the skin in moist areas. The organisms may contribute to the inflammatory component of acne. *Corynebacterium* maximize in the high moisture areas, and like to congregate in the axilla and interdigital skin of the foot. In contrast to *S. aureus*, which is found on only 20% of people, *S. epidermis* is uniformly present on the normal skin. The huge numbers of this resident flora exerts a suppressive effect on other organisms wishing to colonize.

Anaerobic staphylococci are also constantly present. However, they have population densities well below that of other resident flora and unlike other staphylococci do not increase in numbers in dermatologic disease. Gram-negative organisms such as *E. Coli*, Proteus, and Enterobacter are uncommon on normal human skin except in moist intertriginous (skin touching skin) areas, such as toe webs, axillae, and groins. When skin bacteria breaks down the natural secretions from the sebaceous, sweat, and apocrine glands, body odor occurs. Washing with soap and water helps.

In contrast, transient flora act as if they have been deposited from the environment or as fallout from mucous membranes. Aerobic spore formers such as *Bacillus*, various streptococci, and *Neiseria* may briefly visit. Specific ecologic data is difficult to obtain due to sampling data and the transitory changes that occur in each part of our skin.

So-called opportunistic pathogens, bacteria and fungi are generally nonpathogenic members of the resident or transient flora, but can trigger infections in debilitated or compromised hosts. In conditions when the skin is immunocompromised, such as in severe eczema, secondary infection by *Staphylococcus aureus* is common.

Skin disease due to *S. aureus* is the most common of all bacterial infections. Impetigo, with its characteristic yellow crusts and transient vesiculation, and folliculitis, which is a circumscribed infectious process originating in a hair follicle, are generally the most superficial of all staphylococcal skin infections. Tiny red pustules congregate around hair follicles. When the infection is recurrent and chronic in the beard area it is called *sycosis barbae*. Furunculosis (boils) occurs either from an antecedent folliculitis or as deep-seated nodule around a hair follicle. More than 1.5 million cases of furunculosis occur annually in the US alone.

Our tissues are particularly vulnerable to infection in the operating theatre, especially in those patients undergoing extended surgeries such as hip joint replacements. *S. aureus* and other opportunistic bacteria can flourish in a wound with invasion infecting from the patient's own bacteria. However, the primary concern in hospitals is cross-infection by resistant organisms.

Although Anthony van Leeuwenhoek discovered bacteria in the 17th century, it was two centuries before Louis Pasteur linked their existence to disease in *Homo sapiens*. (Incidentally, following his discovery Pasteur suffered from a morbid fear of dirt and infections; he avoided shaking hands for fear of a contamination.) Pasteur also helped to create the world in which cleanliness was next to godliness, which has evolved into a religious zeal displayed incessantly on our television screens: how the death of germs and their byproducts by disinfectants, deodorants, sprays, and cleaning chemicals became a religion, proselytized nightly on the television at enormous costs. But perhaps with a little knowledge, we may find the presence of germs on skin might not be so terrible.

Although when we envision life on the skin as the creeping and hopping evident in larger creatures, the huge majority of our fellow travelers of our own private zoological gardens, numerically, are harmless or beneficial. Each of us supports billions of creatures; since no one can escape from our animal origins it is wise to understand what is happening. Just as we have only begun to explore the undersea world and outer space, the world of our skin is still a great mystery. Our skin is an ecosystem and carries with it all the same issues as the rivers and forests: self-sustaining boundaries, competitive forces for food and growth, and intimate interconnections between itself and resident and transient flora. When a person takes a broad-spectrum antibiotic such as tetracycline, he or she does so with the risk that the diverse set of microclimates of our ecosystem will suffer from imbalance. Our skins have no seasons or diurnal variation and comparatively limited temperature ranges, but have the same complexity and need for ecological integrity of many ecosystems. And given adequate nutrition and care, the skin has tremendous self-healing powers.

> All the wise world is little else, in Nature,
> But parasites or sub-parasites.
> (Ben Jonson, *Volpone*, 1606)

Every move you make results in showers of skin particles released into the air. Every 24 hours an estimated 10,000 million skin scales (or squames) peel off each of our bodies, accounting for 1–1½ grams of skin a day, or about one pound every year. The squames are the desiccated remnants of skin cells that continually form at the base of the epidermis and travel slowly outwards. After 40–56 days a newly formed cell reaches the surface. It has died from the formation of keratin fibres, the same horny components of our hair and finger-nails, and is called the *stratum corneum*. The dead cells are closely attached to each other to form what we call our skin.

At high magnification this surface dead skin appears as irregular patches of curling rough and curly cornflakes. House dust consists of 80–90% skin; squames are the motes in the sunbeams filtering into our rooms.

Viruses are the smallest live inhabitants of our skins and can only reproduce by entering a living cell and fooling it into making more of their own genetic material. The viruses multiply inside the captive cell until it bursts, releasing more virus to colonize other cells. When we have any lowering of our resistance – an infection, sunburn, or stress – the Herpes virus *hominis* that brings on "cold sores" may step into the picture. The virus, which usually begins in childhood, may appear on the skin and then return to the underlying nerves, ebbing and flowing, based on the individual's immunity. Once infected, the virus is carried for life, and more than 90% of the population carry the Herpes virus.

What of the future?

We may have skin detective agencies utilizing bacteriological forensic techniques, pointing to individuals at the scene of a crime. Perhaps the characteristic microflora of a suspect could be just as important to the detective as a fingerprint or other genetic markers. If an individual's microflora, established shortly after birth, remains comparatively constant throughout life, a microbial sampling of room dust, saliva and so on, might reveal groups of identifiable organisms which would match the pattern of a suspect. The particular manner of acquisition of the many different phage-types of bacteria from mother, hospital and early contacts could differentiate two suspects who would support different organisms. By sophisticated phage-typing methods, bacteria could be called to give evidence in court.

Michael Andrew wrote in his book *The Life That Lives on Man*:

> Wherever man goes he is not alone. Though we may
> leave the Earth we take with us on any voyage of
> discovery our own personal world which is yet to be
> completely explored. We evolved on Earth, but we did
> so in the company of the minute creatures which live out
> their lives on our bodies. We should treat our fellow
> travellers with respect; they are much more adaptable
> than we are, and they do us more good than harm.

Perhaps the old adage about "what you don't see can't hurt
you" applies. The huge majority or those critters that live on
the skin are invisible and earn our indifference. And when it
does bother us, at least we have treatments. As far as I know,
we are the only species to have dermatologists, and nail
salons, and beauty parlors, and a myriad of other sources to
rid our body of real or perceived ailments. I am forever
humbled, for along with my fellow soldiers who fight these
ever-lasting skin diseases, I know we can never win the
battle. However, I still choose to fight, to provide
momentary solace from the onslaught of our own invaders,
for the scale-infested sago, and the thousands of patients like
Theresa I treat with skin infestations every year.

Eleven

THE BIRTHMARK REVISITED

In Nathaniel Hawthorne's short story *The Birthmark* (1846) the mad scientist Alymer uses an elixir to remove a miniscule birthmark from the face of his beautiful wife Georgiana.

> "Aylmer," resumed Georgiana, solemnly, "I know not what may be the cost to both of us to rid me of this fatal birthmark. Perhaps its removal may cause cureless deformity; or it may be the stain goes as deep as life itself. Again: do we know that there is a possibility, on any terms, of unclasping the firm grip of this little hand which was laid upon me before I came into the world?"
>
> "Dearest Georgiana, I have spent much thought upon the subject," hastily interrupted Aylmer. "I am convinced of the perfect practicability of its removal."

Hawthorne noted Aylmer's love for his wife to be "intertwined with his love of science." (p 203) He described a young scientist who killed his own wife by pursuing "perfect future" (p 220). Perhaps Aylmer loved science even more than his own wife and to sacrifice her life for a perfect look on her face – for "perfect science" – was a justifiable step. In his obsessive insecurity, Aylmer invests in a need for perfect order in everything, including his wife's face. He lives the ultimate power trip in seeking control and, when the procedure to remove the birthmark results in his wife's death, he becomes the ultimate loser.

If only Aylmer had a trace of empathy instead of an inexorable drive to project his own obstinate pathology onto his wife. In the end Aylmer can find no redemption for his own guilt, and finds himself paradoxically looking into a forever flawed image of his life with the loss of his wife Georgiana.

I believe the book does not demonstrate that Hawthorne was against science; just that he was against "perfect science," and against people like Aylmer who could not separate himself from his science. Hawthorne portrays the idea that nature is equal for everyone because there is no perfection in nature. He writes, "Nature, in one shape or another, stamps ineffaceably on all her productions" (p 205). Georgiana was a beautiful woman, and the birthmark on her face was what kept her in a perpetual balance with nature. Hawthorne shows that any attempt to remove it should and would result in disaster. It is the ultimate cautionary tale: nature, in all its randomness, can only be changed or altered at a price.

But what price should be paid to even attempt perfection, and who should determine it?

Hawthorne saw in his era's fascination with scientific methods, apparatus, and experiments an arrogant temptation, not to learn more about the world and to improve it, but to play God. He also saw how important technology and science were to become to us.

I have often daydreamed while in front of the keyboard about the not too distant future of the dermatologist. In the consulting room advanced technological devices are hooked up into every electrical orifice. Patients come and go, often in less time than it takes a laser beam to penetrate a tattoo.

While the dermatologists of the future are basking in the light of their computer screens, teledermatology will have taken over much of direct patient care. (The new slogan – "If you were a dermatologist, you could be home by now.") Meanwhile pharmacists and mid-level practitioners will be providing vaccine injections for skin cancers and most other dermatological diseases.

In a little known dermatobiblical passage, it is written, "wrinkles are filled, knowledge fades." Remember all your years spent examining and studying the human body, weaving intricate tapestries of shave-sharp therapeutic acumen and piecing together patterns of signs and symptoms? What about all the years our predecessors spent with direct patient care and wrote down their findings? Us dermatologists are the handmaidens of researchers, who have diligently struggled so that we can jot down remedies on prescription pads and get free CDs at medical meetings. The respect and honor for our profession and those that have provided for us may soon fade under the crunch of technology's tyres.

When dermatologists can no longer differentiate a Malphigian from a melanocyte, their differential diagnosis skills atrophied, fading into distant reservoirs in their cerebral cortexes that slowly dry up under the cosmetic sun; when they have all become advanced estheticians with limited academic foundations to serve as a springboard for intellectual endeavors; when the creeping knowledge that their fundamental skills have evaporated like yesterday's cryotherapy spray; after their brains are too scrambled with the selling points of their lotions and creams and snake oils; when they can't tolerate being on the ephemeral see-saw of what is cosmetically fashionable; when the fact that their upcoming laser machine bills are coming due gains purchase in their mind, perhaps they will awaken to the fact that their inner Aylmer has taken over.

Aylmer looks at nature and sees not beauty or symmetry, but imperfections that must be corrected. From a human perspective nature can seem very imperfect: from the blight on our plants to birth defects in our children. We abhor the ravages of disease or the devastating effects of natural disasters. Our first impulse is to do something about them, if the ability to do so lies within our power.

Likewise, Georgiana's birthmark mocks Aylmer, because as a scientist he should be able to do something

about it, to make his wife absolutely flawless. And perhaps
if she were flawless – if he could fix her birthmark today,
her wrinkles tomorrow, her arthritis or cardiac disease forty
years from now....

With his faith in science Aylmer deemed himself
competent to fight against nature and to remove the
birthmark:

> "I feel myself fully competent to render this dear cheek
> as faultless as its fellow; and the, most beloved, what
> will be my triumph when I shall have corrected what
> Nature left imperfect in her fairest work!" (p 207)

But the invasive procedure in pursuit of perfection is
dangerous and, finally, Georgiana is lost. "The crimson
hand, which at first had been strongly visible upon the
marble paleness of Georgiana's cheek, now grew more
faintly outlined. She remained not less pale than ever; but
the birthmark with every breath that came and went, lost
somewhat of its former distinctness. Its presence had been
awful; its departure was more awful still. Watch the stain of
the rainbow fading out the sky, and you will know how that
mysterious symbol passed away."

All becomes clear when we see that it is Georgiana
herself that is the imperfection. As human beings we are
flawed; it is as much a part of our nature as beauty is.
Certainly Aylmer does not consciously recognize that the
inevitable cost of eradicating the imperfection would be to
eradicate Georgiana, but nonetheless that birthmark
symbolizes her very human life. Hawthorne's story
illustrates the sin of overextending our reach from the realm
of the natural into that of the divine.

The modern media continues the portrayal of this never-
ending pursuit of perfection, with television commercials
like giant waterfalls of brainwashing in which viewers can
be swept down into a delusional whirlpool. The eternal

pursuit of the unattainable is presented nightly – perfect health if only you use a certain drug or hygiene product or ingest a particular food or drink. The television show *Nip/Tuck* perhaps epitomizes the current perfection-seeking story. It is a cautionary tale of two unscrupulous Miami plastic surgeons and boatloads of neurotic patients who are searching desperately for surgical cures for their insatiable unhappiness. Other TV shows have fed the national obsession for eternal youth, including the reality show *Extreme Makeover* in which dished out liposuction and nose jobs to ordinary people, but *Nip/Tuck* has continued to feed the powerful delusion of the baby-boomer generation in the most graphic way, with breast augmentations, buttock implants and hot sex scenes, all performed to the tune of pounding rock music.

In each episode of this dark satire the consultations begin with the plastic surgeon requesting, "Tell me what you don't like about yourself." One of the patients, an aspiring model, states, "I don't want to be pretty. I want to be better ... I want to be perfect." However, the showcased talented surgeons rarely improve lives with their nips, tucks, and more aggressive procedures, let alone save them.

I have often turned away potential patients that have "image issues". Red flags rise high when I talk with those who are requesting procedures to please someone other than themselves; those who have ideals of social perfectionism; those with the morbid dissatisfaction of body dysmorphic syndrome or other deep emotional scars, or those who just have generally unrealistic expectations. Botox and chemical peels may improve your sense of self-esteem but it rarely saves a floundering marriage.

There are patients who don't want cosmetic procedures and have the commonsense to not always look for medical cures for their unhappiness. Often they have real medical concerns – skin cancers, horrible acne, or miserable psoriasis. I am not a cosmetic Luddite – I've botoxed a few rhytides and made leg telangiectasias disappear – but everything in moderation and with care. Dermatology's medical knowledge should separate and elevate us from those scurrying around in every Fountain of Youth Clinic of Cosmetics in the country.

What have our great teachers written on the subject of perfection?

In Section VII, number 87, the last aphorism of Hippocrates, he writes, "Those diseases which medicines do not cure, iron [the knife] cures; those which iron cannot cure, fire cures; and those which fire cannot cure, are to be reckoned wholly incurable." That is to say, some things are better left alone.

Hippocrates also wrote, "Life is short, and Art long; the crisis fleeting; experience perilous, and decision difficult." No one ever said it was going to be easy, and attempts at perfection are frivolous.

In the book *Nature's Chaos*, written by James Gleick with photographs by the physician/photographer Eliot Porter (2001), Gleick writes, "The essence of the earth's beauty lies in disorder, a peculiarly patterned disorder, from the fierce tumult of rushing water to the filigrees of unbridled vegetation." I submit that the essence of human beauty also lies in its unpredictability, a pathology that draws our divine attention, an irreverent, captivating punch line almost imperceptibly delivered.

We have plowed ahead in the field of cosmetic surgery, trying to discover a remedy for every one of life's built-in deformities, rarely pausing to question the price in both economic and life quality terms. As Dr Ian Malcom (played by Jeff Goldblum) states in the movie *Jurassic Park*, "We were so busy finding out if we could that we never stopped to find out if we should."

Twelve

NOT A WOLF

A 28-year-old African-American woman named Annie B. was on the examining table pointing to the lesions on her face. I looked closer and noted eroded areas on the sides of her face and scalp that looked like miniature grenades had exploded and left crevices.

"How long have these been there?" I asked.

"A couple of years. But now they are getting worse."

In addition, she had a red, raised rash that spread across her cheeks, the bridge of her nose, and above her eyes.

I looked over the history section in her chart for medications. None were listed.

"So you don't take any prescription or other medications?"

"Nope. Just a bunch of aspirin or whatever I can afford because my bones ache."

I had my suspicions and now I had to put them to the test.

I performed a small punch biopsy of one of the lesions. I ordered a full blood count to detect anemia, low platelets or low white bloodcells; creatinine and electrolytes to measure the salts in the blood and kidney function; a urinalysis to measure protein and bloodcells in urine or to identify 'casts' (blobs of protein escaped from the bloodstream because the kidneys are leaky), and blood clotting tests, liver function tests, and an ESR (Erythrocyte Sedimentation Rate) – a marker of non-specific inflammation, and the CRP (C-reactive protein) – another inflammatory marker, and an Anti-Nuclear Antibody (ANA) test.

As the results rolled in and I gathered more facts, the diagnostic picture cleared. The CRP was normal and the ANA was positive. Along with the results of the biopsy, the lab results led me to her diagnosis – systemic lupus erythematosus. The positive ANA test, when found in the blood when the patient is not taking drugs, is known as a positive test for lupus in most cases, but it is not necessarily conclusive. Other components are required to complete the picture.

What is systemic lupus erythematosus?

Normally, when our body is under attack by viruses and bacteria, white bloodcells in our immune system, known as B cells, respond by producing antibodies to help fight off the foreign invaders. Antibodies bind to these invaders, inactivate them, and mark them for destruction. Lupus, however, is an autoimmune disease, and the ability to discriminate between self-molecules and foreign invaders is broken down. Lupus allows B cells to produce antibodies that attack healthy cells and tissues, including vital organs.

In addition to arthritis, facial rash, and hair loss, other manifestations of lupus include kidney damage, lung inflammation, and paralysis. Many other diseases can mimic systemic lupus erythematosus, such as scleroderma – a hardening of the skin caused by overproduction of collagen, multiple sclerosis, characterized by fatigue, heaviness or clumsiness in the arms and legs, rheumatoid arthritis, or myositis. Lupus is therefore a difficult disease to diagnose and can be overlooked, often for years. Another patient of mine appeared to have either severe acne scars or self-induced scars from "nervous picking," but with further exploration I discovered that she, too, had lupus.

Approximately 90% of lupus sufferers are women; most develop the disease during their childbearing years. Lupus accounts for more than 100,000 hospital admissions in the US each year, averaging 10 days and about $20,000 per visit. Lupus patients lose between 30 and 100 work days per year.

The American College of Rheumatology requires that someone with a diagnosis of lupus must have at least 4 of 11 manifestations at any time since the onset of the disease. Annie B had fit that criterion, having had the "butterfly" or "red wolf" mark, the eroded red patches of skin, pain in the joints, and a positive ANA test.

Lupus unfortunately has poor treatment options and there have been no real recent advancements in therapy. Treatment with corticosteroids and chemotherapy drugs has significantly increased 10-year patient survival rates. However, these drugs remain a principal cause of morbidity and mortality in lupus. Until effective non-toxic treatments for lupus exist, people like Annie have to settle for what we can offer. Most current approaches address only disease symptoms and provide non-specific treatments that suppress the overall immune system, killing healthy B cells and leaving the patient susceptible to serious infections.

As Annie had developed various cutaneous symptoms, I treated her with topical cortisones and intralesional steroids to reduce her inflammation. I sent her to a rheumatologist who put her on oral steroids and other therapies. Annie understood it was a chronic disease with acute exacerbations, or "flares," but, like most people, found it difficult to come to grips with why she had "come down with this."

Over the next several months Annie and I discussed many of the problems she was struggling with as a result of her lupus. "I don't like this on my face," she said, pointing to the red rash. The infamous "butterfly" rash is a classic feature of lupus. This rash has also been called the "red wolf" mark, for which the disease is named.

Annie shook her head in irritation. "People ask me everything from 'What did you get on your face?' to 'What the heck happened to your face?'"

When she had a flare her frustration heightened. "I look and feel bad," she said. "And now I'm losing my hair." I examined a few small areas of alopecia, which had left bald, red, rashy patches in place of scalp hair.

"And I'm growing hair where I don't want to. I wish I could take it and plant it in my scalp." (A side effect of long-term steroid use is an increase of body hair, mostly on the upper lips, forearms and chin.)

I recommended her to an excellent beautician and esthetician for her hair problems. A good cut and style could do wonders and for the patchy kind of alopecia from which Annie was suffering; hair swatches or even full-head wigs can help. Special make-up can be applied, such as the kind that burn patients can use to help diminish the appearance of scars. And the esthetician can also help get rid of unwanted hair.

"And I can't get my ring off my finger." I looked at her hands and saw evidence of edema, or water retention, which can also occur with steroids.

"What else?" I asked.

"I don't like all these weight changes," she said. "It's hard to shop when my dress size keeps going up and down."

"What's happening?" I asked.

"Some days I can't eat because I'm sick to my stomach. And people keep asking what's wrong with me. And then when I went on the steroids I gained weight. And I get restless, can't get to sleep, and get all worn out looking. I know I need the medicines, but sometimes I don't even want to look in the mirror."

Chemotherapy medications have inherent side effects in many lupus patients. A fine balance exists with long-term use of steroids, which can lead to Cushing's syndrome. Fat can be redistributed to the face ("moon face"), the upper back and shoulders ("hump back" or "buffalo hump"), and the abdomen, creating a "top heavy" look. Good nutrition and exercise are helpful in controlling weight.

Other possible problems associated with lupus include photosensitivity rash after exposure to sunlight, small sores that occur in mucosal lining of mouth and nose, inflammation of the delicate tissues covering internal organs and abdominal pain, seizures or psychosis, anemia and other blood disorders.

Kidney disease occurs in half of lupus patients and is a leading cause of morbidity and mortality. Life-threatening episodes of kidney inflammation can require expensive intensive-care hospitalization. Kidney dialysis costs more than $40,000 per year in the US.

Deterioration and loss of hip and knee joints can occur as a result of the side effects of high-dose corticosteroid therapy. Hip replacement surgery, which may be required, costs about $30,000 per hip operation. Treatments with high doses of immunosuppressive drugs can result in severe adverse side effects such as diabetes, hypertension, psychosis, cataracts, and sterility. On top of all that is the vulnerable psyche of the lupus patient.

"Some days it feels like it's my fault. I get real down and feel guilty."

I offered Annie what I could. Perhaps most important were our talks about her frustrations with the disease. I wish I could make the wolf scoot into the woods, leaving the calm face of someone who never deserved to be co-inhabited.

Thirteen

APOLLO'S LEGACY

When I walked in the room to introduce myself to Guillermo, I knew he represented a challenge of long duration. Populating his face and neck were at least 15 easily recognizable skin cancers spread out in odd arrangements and patterns. He had one of the worst collective cases of these cancers that I had ever seen. None of them were immediately life threatening, but the disfigurement was horrible. "I have most of these many years," he said in broken English. "My family tell me I need to get them off."

"Your family is right," I said.

Guillermo had spent his first 50 years in Cuba, a country with a disturbing record for skin cancer prevention. In my own small sampling, many of my worst skin cancer patients have been from Cuba. However, the skin cancer prevention program is not much better in the United States. According to the National Cancer Institute, approximately 40–50% of Americans who live to the age of 65 will have skin cancer at least once.

And Guillermo had not fared much better in the US either. Arriving in Florida five years ago, he had exchanged one tropical country for another, and he had done little to protect himself from further skin insult and injury.

Kurt Vonnegut was asked to be the guest speaker for a prestigious college's commencement exercise, and this is the first and last portion of what he told the graduating class:

> "Wear sunscreen. If I could offer you only one tip for the future, sunscreen would be it. The long-term benefits of sunscreen have been proved by scientists, whereas the rest of my advice has no basis more reliable than my own meandering experience. [...] Advice is a form of

nostalgia. Dispensing it is a way of fishing the past from the disposal, wiping it off, painting over the ugly parts and recycling it for more than it's worth. But trust me on the sunscreen."

During my childhood summers in Michigan, where I grew up a distance less than an hour from the beach, I had cherished the sun. I recall the smell of baby oil mixed in with the thin toasty smell of heated skin. I savored the precious two months of the year when I could actually lay in the sun with scant clothing; the memories of giant snow piles melting to my mind's periphery. Now, as an adult I have to worry about what I had thought of as a benevolent sun being some type of malicious nuclear reactor that has melted down my skin and turned my DNA into a skin cancer-making machine. I need to add eternal vigilance about the devastating effects of the sun to all the other problems of our day-to-day life – the threat of terrorism, Lyme disease, West Nile virus and long lines at Dunkin' Donuts. And, as a dermatologist, I have to help others heed that wake-up call.

The first Greek sun god was Helios. We use the term dermatoheliosis in reference to photoaging or sun damage on the skin. Later Apollo became the accepted sun god. Apollo was also the god of healing and prophecy. Aesculapius, Apollo's mortal son, was said to be the first physician, and his staff entwined by a serpent is used as Western medicine's symbol.

Over 400 years ago, Copernicus declared the sun as the center of our universe. The healing power of the sun has always been evident: from cave dwellers worshiping the sun to the sun's germicidal powers and ability to diminish various skin diseases such as psoriasis. Vitamin D synthesis and the feel-good effects of the sun (an antidote to seasonal affective disorder for those in dreary Northern climates) also play major roles in our love of the sun. But perhaps not even Apollo could foresee the sun's damaging effects on future generations.

How did this oceanic change in our sense of what the sun means to us come about?

Much of the history of sun tanning carries with it a media hype akin to that for cigarette smoking. During the 1920s and 1930s, many movie stars were paid to smoke at prime attention-getting locations, thus enabling the tobacco companies to increase their sales dramatically. In similar ways, the Coco Chanels of the world launched huge media and tanning spikes. Betty Grable, Rita Hayworth, and other bathing beauties were pictured in one- and two-piece bathing suits exposing their tanned bodies. European women sun-bathed in decorative, ostentatious sunhats and shawls for fashionable reasons, not for protection. And if their skin happened to have any spot without a tan, brown and beige tinted powders and creams were available. The fashion industry created shoes to be worn without stockings and sleeveless dresses for women wanting to expose their tans. And a tan in winter was a clear sign that the tan bearer had enough wealth and leisure to afford to holiday in an exotic, warm climate.

In 1929 Helena Reubenstein warned, "sunburn menaces your beauty." The ingredient PABA (para-aminobenzoic acid) was introduced in sunscreen products in 1943. But while the public ambiguity about the pale or tanned look persisted, women's magazines encouraged sun lamps and tanning, and cosmetic companies introduced sun-tanning oils. Certain science reporters used women's magazines to suggest that gradual tanning could cancel out the sun's harmful skin damaging effects. *Harper's Bazaar*, in 1954, reported, "There are sunscreen preparations that can cut the intensity of the sun's rays by 75%." But the media slowly accepted the message about the serious damage that sun can do to the skin.

In my medical practice, there is not a week that goes by when someone does not say to me, "We didn't know about the problem with the sun when we were younger." They clearly may not have known about it, but it was evident in the media.

Tanned skin became a status symbol in the 1960s. Coppertone advertisements filled the airwaves – "Tan, don't burn. Get a Coppertone tan!" – and beach movies filled with bikini-clad teens populated the television. In the 1970s, with gallons of baby oil coating many an unsuspecting epidermis, another industry began to blossom – the indoor tanning industry. Now, even those in the cold North could try to keep a tan or prepare for adventures to warmer climates with a series of trips to the tanning salon.

But, in addition to the cancer-producing and premature wrinkling effects of the sun, self-tanning units emitted high levels of UVB light that burned the skin and didn't tan. More advanced tanning units emitted both UVB and UVA rays and brought on further damage. The tanning industry, almost entirely unregulated, continued to prosper.

In the early 1970s the FDA began to treat sunscreens as over-the-counter drugs rather than cosmetics, so more stringent labeling was required. After the FDA began regulating sunscreens, the maker's of Johnson's Baby Oil warned that the heroine of their ads should "take a little less sun." In 1978 the FDA declared sunscreens to be safe, effective, and useful in preventing skin cancer and sunburn, and slowing down premature aging of the skin. The SPF numbering system was developed using numbers 2-15.

By the mid-1980s, public education program about the dangers of overexposure to the sun and the problems associated with self-tanning began to grow. The American Academy of Dermatology voiced its strong support of sun protection, and sunscreen manufacturers produced higher SPF products.

Malignant melanoma studies showed a 500% increase from 1950 to 1985. A 1987 American Academy of Dermatology study revealed that 96% of Americans admitted to knowing that the sun caused skin cancer. But one third of the adults in the survey admitted they deliberately worked on a tan.

The indoor tanning industry continued to be one of the fastest growing businesses in America. The average age of indoor tanning patrons was 26, mostly women. Almost two million of these patrons were considered "tanning junkies", making almost 100 tanning parlor visits per year. In 1991, 1,800 injuries were reported from the use of tanning devices.

By the late 1980s fashion industry leaders such as Eileen Ford stated, "The tanned look is dead." The American Academy of Dermatology stated that there was "no safe way to tan" following a consensus conference on photoaging and photodamage (in reality, a tan is simply a controlled burn). Wide ranges of protection against UVA as well as UVB radiation were created by the sunscreen industry in 1990 in response to the rising tide of information about skin cancer facts – 600,000 new cases of skin cancers, 6,300 deaths from melanoma and 2,500 deaths from squamous cell carcinoma. The role of genetics, ozone depletion, and other skin cancer production factors took center stage.

The incidence of skin cancer continued to increase throughout the 1990s, with 700,000 new cases of skin cancer diagnosed in 1993, 32,000 of them malignant melanoma. A survey in 1996 of young adults under 25 indicated 58% of them confessed to working on a tan and 62% that they thought people looked better with a tan. In 1997, a survey in *Seventeen* magazine stated that two thirds of teenagers felt they looked better with a tan and felt healthier and more sophisticated. Half of them stated they looked more athletic with a tan. Although more than half the states in the US had rules and regulations for tanning salons, the tanning industry grew to almost 20,000 tanning salons in America with 22 million customers per year. The American Academy of Dermatology continued to warn the public that they should minimize the sun's damage to the skin and eyes by planning outdoor activities to avoid the sun's strongest rays, wearing protective covering, wearing sunglasses and always wearing a broad spectrum sunscreen.

The waves of history lap onto the shores of today. The unprotected sun exposures of all these earlier generations are now causing a bloom of skin cancers. We, as dermatologists, use whatever mechanisms are necessary to rid our patients of skin cancers at all stages of development. We sprint around looking for ways to prevent and treat these by chemoprevention, radiation, laser, cryotherapy, and surgical excisions. We are the gardeners of the skin, but cancers sprout up everywhere like unrestricted weeds. We are like children during a summer shower trying to catch all the raindrops in our cups knowing that so many fall to the ground. We can only get rid of what we can see and, therefore, we urge our patients and explain in the media the importance of skin cancer prevention, detection and treatment.

I know it is difficult to get people to change their behavior, but prevention really is better than cure. Sunscreens with protection factor 15 and higher have been readily available since the early 1980s and, of course, they are available today in a variety of topical preparations. I certainly preach the gospel of using sunscreens, especially to the parents of vulnerable children, which will pay off in huge cost savings and treatment prevention in future years. I regularly see patients in their twenties and thirties with skin cancers, and in the last two years have had a 14- and a 15-

year-old in my office presenting with stage IV malignant melanomas.

But what were my options with Guillermo?

He had the wrong kind of insurance to allow for advanced surgeries and not enough money to pay for anything cosmetic. With his consent I chose to perform a series of shave biopsies and electrodessications and to allow his healing skin to do the rest. "I am very happy to get better," he said. Over time he improved, exchanging skin cancers for scars – a trade-off that occurs thousands of times a day throughout the world that Apollo once ruled.

Fourteen

FROM DRACULA TO CANCER SLAYER

"I've got these blisters that hurt like crazy," my patient said, and pointed to the painful blisters on the backs of his hands.

My patient, 47-year-old Richard, was a roofer and said the blisters had come out "since the warm weather had begun." He denied any recent exposure to poison ivy or sumac, new soaps or detergents, or to new medications. He also did not complain of chills or fevers, previous episodes of blistering, or lesions in his mouth. He did say, "My pee looks different." I asked him what he meant and he reported a reddish-orange tint. He admitted to an average daily ethanol intake of about 8 12-oz cans of beer and smoking a pack of cigarettes per day.

The dorsal surfaces of both of Richard's hands and forearms were covered with numerous intact and ruptured bullae, with areas of erosion. His face and neck were covered with the thickly wrinkled, hyperpigmented skin of chronic solar elastosis.

Many blistering diseases needed to be considered, including herpetic infections or staphylococcal infection. A 3-mm punch biopsy of a bulla showed findings of porphyria. Richard had porphyria cutanea tarda.

Porphyria is a rare disorder filled with all the drama of a compelling disease – misanthropic enzyme pathways, heightened sensitivities, and a fascinating history. Porphyria comprises seven separate disorders, and the rarest form – congenital erythropoietic porphyria – causes severe disfigurement. Photosensitivity is the hallmark of porphyria cutanea tarda. Ultraviolet light transforms accumulated porphyrins in the skin into toxins that cause skin fragility. The dorsal surfaces of the hands are the principal sites of bullae formation because of exposure to sun and trauma.

Shortly after the bullae form, they rupture and become painful erosions that heal as atrophic scars and milia.

Porphyrias result from inherited or acquired deficiencies in any one of several enzymes that synthesize heme. If a given enzyme is absent or in short supply, porphyrins are shunted away from heme synthesis into pathways that produce porphyrin byproducts. These byproducts build up in tissues and cause the clinical manifestations of porphyria.

Porphyria also has a fascinating history tied in with tales of Dracula and other bloodsuckers.

Bram Stoker's vampire novel *Dracula* is one of the most popular novels of all time. It was an immediate success when first published in London in 1897 and has remained in print ever since. Films, stage adaptations, comic books, and even a ballet have brought the story of the loathsome blood-sucking vampire count to a worldwide audience in the millions.

The novel draws on the historical belief in frightening vampire creatures. The vampire is noted in the literatures of ancient Egypt and Greece, but *Dracula* – set in Transylvania, a wild, rocky region in the Carpathian Mountains – borrows most deeply from the folk beliefs of rural Romania.

The Eastern Orthodox Church – the dominant religion in Romania – proclaimed that people who died under a curse or a ban of excommunication would become walking dead, or "moroi," until granted absolution by the church. In addition, local superstition added creatures known as "strigoi," demon birds that fly only at night, greedy for human flesh and blood. It was also believed that those dying from plague became weak from loss of blood; and an early folk remedy for the loss of hemoglobin (which contains a porphyrin) may have been to drink blood. In extreme cases of porphyria, the victim's lips and gums erode to reveal red, fanglike teeth.

Garlic can exacerbate an attack. And so we have all the elements of vampirism and its accompanying stories.

Romanian legends suggest that certain individuals, such as illegitimate or unbaptized children, witches, and the seventh son of a seventh son, are doomed to become vampires. In some villages anyone who refused to eat garlic was suspected of being a vampire. Protection from night assaults by the drinkers of blood was best assured by rubbing garlic on all windows and doors.

For those of you familiar with the novel, you will recall that Count Dracula travels to England to spread his vampire cult. However, he is eventually foiled when Jonathan Harker, the young hero, escapes from the castle and joins forces with Dr Abraham Van Helsing, a Dutch expert on vampirism. Helsing and Harker discover that Dracula cannot endure sunlight, garlic, or the symbol of the Christian cross, and can be killed only with a stake driven through the heart.

In the 1970s, in a truly horrendous crime, 28-year-old Richard Chase, the "Dracula Killer," murdered Evelyn Miroth and Daniel Meredith in Sacramento, California. He removed some of the organs of Miroth's body and filled them with blood before taking them with him. Chase was tracked down and found in a field, naked and covered in cow's blood. Apparently, Chase had porphyria and his behavior did not come as a complete surprise to those who knew him. As a child, he had reportedly killed many animals, drinking the blood of a bird on one occasion.

Chase had been in and out of psychiatric hospitals for most of his life; a year prior to the killings, Chase was released because his psychiatrist found that Chase had a handle on his problems. Police found that Chase's home was filled with human blood, in the blender and in the sinks, suggesting that Chase had been drinking it for some time.

In 1979, Chase went to trial; his attorney arguing in his defense that he was insane and had a chemical disorder that made him drink blood. The jury found him sane and sentenced him to life in prison. On the day after Christmas in 1980, Chase killed himself in his cell at San Quentin.

In the mid 1980s, medical accounts of the extremely rare disease porphyria (only 60 cases have been reported) brought on speculation about the possible basis for the vampire legends. Electrifying press accounts made much of the "Dracula disease." As noted, only congenital erythropoietic porphyria produces serious disfigurement and the "Vampire-like" characteristics: pointed teeth, excessive hair, extreme sensitivity to light, and the need for blood. However, the journalistic accounts of the medical research on porphyria proved once again that public fascination with the fictional Dracula remains intact, echoing the young Harker's question in the novel: "What manner of man is this, or what manner of creature is it in the semblance of man?"

Now Dracula has been killed and the ancient superstitions hopefully have diminished (generations of Romanian children have been threatened with the folk warning, "Be good, or Dracula will get you"). Today, however, we have our own terrifying parasitic creature that threatens to "get us" – cancer. And porphyria has played an important role in the development of treatments for cancer, as well as other diseases.

Photodynamic therapy (PDT) received a standing ovation when Nick Lane, an honorary research fellow at University College London, wrote an article in *Scientific American*, stating that PDT "has grown from an improbable treatment for cancer in the 1970s to a sophisticated and effective weapon against a diverse array of malignancies today."

The inspiration for PDT was a result of research into porphyria. In the mid-20th century scientists hypothesized that the toxic effects of light-sensitive porphyrins might be therapeutically quite valuable. As Lane reported, "If a porphyrin is injected into diseased tissue, such as a cancerous tumor, it can be activated by light to destroy that tissue." This remarkable discovery was the origin of PDT as a cancer therapy.

PDT is now also being used as a treatment for age-related macular degeneration and pathologic myopia and experimentally for coronary artery disease, AIDS, autoimmune diseases, transplantation rejection and leukemia.

How does it work?

All porphyrins have in common a flat ring (composed of carbon and nitrogen) with a central hole that provides space for a metal ion to bind to it. If the central atom is iron, the molecule becomes hemoglobin; if it is magnesium, it becomes chlorophyll. (A copper-centered porphyrin, called hemocyanin, gives the blood of horseshoe crabs a blue tint.) Lane calls these substances at the heart of PDT "among the oldest and most important of all biological molecules, because they orchestrate the two most critical energy-generating processes in life: photosynthesis and oxygen respiration." The molecules he is referring to – chlorophyll and hemoglobin – yield, respectively, the "green" and "red" photosensitizing agents we use today.

Photodynamic therapy is based on the therapeutic interaction of light, oxygen, and a photosensitizing agent. When metal-free porphyrins become excited they absorb light at certain wavelengths and their electrons jump into higher-energy orbitals. Says Lane, "The molecules can then transmit their excitation to other molecules having the right kind of bonds, especially oxygen, to produce reactive singlet oxygen and other highly reactive and destructive molecules known as free radicals."

Although free radicals are thought of as uniformly undesirable, they can be used to achieve a desirable destruction inside the dangerous cancer cell. "Metal-free porphyrins are not the agents, but rather the brokers, of destruction," says Lane. "They catalyze the production of toxic forms of oxygen." PDT reflects a trend in oncology away from conventional cytotoxic treatments and towards innovative approaches that are highly selective for cancer.

But what of Richard?

Avoidance of precipitating factors is the cornerstone of treatment for porphyria. Richard was advised to protect himself from ultraviolet light by wearing long sleeves, gloves, and a hat; applying sunscreen with an SPF greater than 15; and changing his occupation to one that is predominantly indoors. He also was counseled to abstain from drinking alcohol (ethanol).

Richard was poorly compliant with the conservative measures; I had tried to instill in him a sense of respect for his disease, but his obedience had fallen short. Phlebotomy was the next appropriate step. 500 mL of blood was removed weekly until his hemoglobin concentration dropped to between 10 and 11 g/dL and his serum iron levels fell to between 50 and 60 micrograms/dL. He has been in clinical remission for the past two years, but in the future he will more than likely need to resume phlebotomy unless he falls off a roof from drinking. As an indefatigable optimist, I hope and pray he will survive to donate his blood once again.

Fifteen

WARTS NEW?

I told the little eight-year-old boy, Ricky Fawcett, that he had warts. What a word! *Warts*.

What are warts?

Warts are common harmless skin growths, which can be an irritation. Warts can grow on any part of the body and their appearance depends on their location – raised on the face and tops of the hands, and thickened and flatter on the soles of the feet (plantar warts) from the pressure of standing. They have a rough surface on which tiny, dark dots can often be seen. Warts can bleed if injured, but common warts never turn cancerous.

What causes warts?

A virus, they are contagious to other areas on the body or to other susceptible children. Plantar warts are also contagious and are frequently picked up in moist areas. The best method of prevention is to keep your feet dry after being in one of these areas such as bathrooms, locker rooms and around swimming pools. Genital and perianal warts are also directly contagious by contact, and care must be taken not to spread them to others.

And what a handful little Ricky had! Or should I say two handfuls – one foot and one on the corner of his mouth.

"I told him not to go out in the woods and play with any frogs," his mother said, totally serious. The number of sincere adults who tell their children, in front of me, not to touch any more frogs amazes me.

But regardless of how someone determines the etiology of the wart, the greatest concern rapidly shifts to their removal. Wart-removing stories collect and hang in the air of my exam rooms on a weekly basis and sometimes I snatch them down and put them on memoir paper. A few of them are mind-numbingly stupid, others just slightly daffy.

Here are some tales.

Get an apple. Cut it into as many pieces as you have warts. Match each apple piece to a wart and rub that piece on the wart. Put the apple back together and bury it. As soon as the apple rots, the warts will be gone! The symbolic removal of a wart by fruit – sympathetic magic!

Tape a piece of banana peel on the wart.

Make the wart bleed. Put one drop of blood on seven grains of corn. Feed the corn to an old black hen.

Tie a human hair around the wart and leave it in place for several days. Remove the hair and place it in a nail hole in a green tree. Replace the nail, driving it into the hair so it will be stuck in the tree. When the hair rots, the wart will disappear.

Rub an old bone on the wart and throw it over your shoulder.

Superstitions and folk remedies for warts also include…

The bacon cure: Two days after the full moon, take a piece of bacon, rub it on your wart, and then bury the bacon. (This same technique is said to work with half a raw potato or nine grains of corn.)

The penny cure: Rub 20 copper pennies on your wart and then give the coins away to someone who needs them. (Obviously, this is a very old remedy, but I admire its altruistic spirit.)

The pebbles cure: Rub your wart with pebbles, put the pebbles in a bag, and toss the bag over your left shoulder. (And make sure nobody is standing behind you.)

The written-wish cure: Write a wish on a piece of paper, carry it to the intersection of two streets, then tear up the paper and scatter it to the four winds. (Beware of the police so you don't get arrested for littering.)

The beans-in-a-bag cure: Put as many beans in a paper bag as you have warts, and place the bag at the intersection of two streets. The next person to pick up the bag will get your warts.

Or have somebody count your warts. Your warts will go away, but the person who counted the growths will get them.

But for the wickedest wart-removal strategy of all, here's the technique that Huckleberry Finn swore by in Mark Twain's book *Tom Sawyer* (1876):

"Take a dead cat to a graveyard where someone wicked has been buried, wait until midnight for the devil to come, then heave your cat at the devil while saying, 'Devil follow corpse, cat follow devil, warts follow cat, I'm done with ye!'"

One of my middle-aged patients told me that the way she got rid of warts when she was a kid was to have them bought from her. Her uncle asked if he could buy the warts for a quarter. He gave her a quarter and the warts were gone in two weeks.

How about breaking open the stem of a dandelion and rubbing the milky sap on the warts in a circular motion? Do this two or three times a day until the wart disappears. (This was the favorite remedy of Will Greer, Grandpa Walton on the TV show *The Waltons*.)

Other reported wart removers include cayenne pepper, garlic, aloe, apple cider vinegar, wood ashes, aspirin, baking soda, or cashews (one patient said he chewed the cashew and took a small amount of the mixture and placed it on the wart to remove a wart he had had for 25 years), castor oil, white chalk, Elmer's® glue, diced garlic, grapefruit seed extract, lemon juice, hydrogen peroxide, iodine, pineapple, onion, papaya, milkweed, potato radish, pokeweed, or turnip. Oral intake of dessicated liver has also been suggested. Homeopathic remedies include Thuja, Causticum, Nitric acid, Antimonium crudum and Berberis.

Duct tape has also been in vogue in recent years. Although if you cover the wart with any kind of medical or first aid tape or a band-aid and leave it on around the clock for three weeks, removing only to change the tape, you may cure the wart.

Common folk remedies for wart removal continue almost endlessly, with witches, toads, buried totems, and bizarre concoctions. No one yet has come up with an instant cure, although people have been trying for thousands of years. Perhaps the "success" of some folk remedies for warts can be linked to the fact that warts often disappear of their own accord, especially in young children. Average clearance time may be as long as two years, but this spontaneous disappearance is less common in older children and adults.

What about hypnosis or guided imagery to rid your skin of warts?

The skin has loads of nerve endings, which act as channels to and from your brain. Many skin disorders – including acne, rashes, and warts – are affected by changes in your mental state, such as mood swings or stress. If a person using superstition, guided imagery, hypnosis or other alternative therapy truly believes they will work, warts are good targets for destruction due to their susceptibility to mind over matter dynamics.

A hypnotherapy treatment may start with the hypnotherapist getting you very relaxed so that you can enter into a "trance" – a state in which your mind is very open to suggestion. Your hypnotherapist may take you on a journey where you imagine traveling inside your body to the roots of your offending growths. Perhaps you'll be told to cut these roots off from nourishment from your body by whatever means your imagination dictates, perhaps by strangling them with a lasso or gently covering them with a destructive paint. After the suggestion is planted in your mind, you'll be told to forget about it.

In a similar vein, I have told hundred of kids to imagine their hands clear from warts every night before they go to bed. Even if it doesn't clear them, I believe it helps. Because most warts will eventually go away on their own anyway, if you time your mind therapy at the proper waning you may be instilling a double-whammy for wart disappearance.

However, home treatment with a salicylic acid preparation is often the first-line treatment for warts. Products with salicylic acid work by destroying wart tissue. The *British Medical Journal* surveyed 50 trials and reported that this remedy cured non-genital warts in 75% of the cases as opposed to 48% using a placebo. A helpful hint: when using salicylic acid preparation, apply it only to the wart, not on the surrounding skin. The basic drill is to apply it twice daily and soak and rub the dead wart tissue away before reapplying. If you get pain or irritation, stop for a few days, then start again. You can apply the salicylic acid with a toothpick or other small applicator if the wart is tiny. If you have warts on the soles of your feet or the palms of your hands you can use salicylic acid plaster.

Although home treatment can be as effective, less expensive and less painful as treatment from your doctor, it may take longer. The salicylic acid in the doctor's office is a more aggressive treatment and produces a controlled burn. Also, you must be certain that a skin growth is a wart. Especially in older patients I have biopsied "warts" that have turned out to be squamous cell carcinomas or other ominous diseases. And if you have diabetes, peripheral vascular disease, or other major illnesses that may affect your treatment, it is best to see a doctor.

Much has been written about the blistering power of cantharidin – a substance derived from the blister beetle that has been used medicinally for more than 2,000 years in China. Cantharidin is found in the body fluids of more than 1,500 species of blister beetle; two species are commonly found in the southern and southwestern United States. The "beetle juice" of the blister beetle (also known as the Spanish fly) has long been infamous as a purported aphrodisiac. However, when taken orally, cantharidin is poisonous and can even be fatal.

In a 2001 article in the *Archives of Dermatology*, researchers from New York University's School of Medicine reviewed 49 studies and articles and took a comprehensive look at cantharidin's origins, folk uses, current FDA status, dermatologic uses, and toxic effects. The article reported that in the 1950s, US dermatologists had used cantharidin to treat warts but the substance lost its FDA approval in 1962 when new manufacturing regulations went into effect. Manufacturers of cantharidin products apparently failed to submit required data. For almost forty years it was lost as a treatment, but a 1997 amendment to the Food, Drug, and Cosmetics Act allowed cantharidin to be nominated for the FDA's Bulk Substances List, which allows physicians to administer drugs compounded with cantharidin and other ingredients.

In cantharidin treatment the physician applies the drug to the wart and a very narrow circle of surrounding skin. The area is sealed with nonporous tape, which is removed after four hours. Cantharidin destroys warts by creating a blister that causes the wart to detach from the surrounding skin, which generally occurs within 24–48 hours. Healing is normally complete within 4–7 days. Resistant warts occasionally will require a second treatment.

Techniques to stimulate the immune system and clear the warts by mimicking the way our body naturally clears warts have recently been introduced. An oral medication that stimulates the immune system has been used for widespread, recalcitrant warts. We are, however, unable to kill the wart virus, and there is no way to prevent warts, although researchers are attempting to solve that problem.

With Ricky, I used cantharidin over three treatments after first painlessly removing (paring down) small sections of the warts to allow deeper penetration of the "beetle juice". I also told him my favorite wart story.

"I am so happy you have given me your warts. I have to feed the monster that lives under the sink a certain amount of warts or he comes out at Hallowe'en and scares the heck out of the kids around town." I quickly opened the cabinet and said, "Stay in there," and shut it fast.

Sixteen

A DAY IN THE LIFE

One of the reasons I like dermatology is because I deal with mostly healthy people on an outpatient basis. In nursing homes, it's a mix. When I did primary care, I always had this sense of there being two types of people: those who are healthy and those who are not and I felt it was my task to find out which of those worlds the person in front of me was in. In fact, we all live in that border world, as Shakespeare wrote in *As You Like It*:

And so from hour to hour we ripe, and ripe,
And then from hour to hour we rot and rot,
And thereby hangs a tale.

The mystery of the primary care patient was intriguing, although exhausting. Was the abdominal pain just a slight upset or the harbinger of gastric cancer? Did the pain in the shoulder reflect bursitis or cardiac pathology? As the information in each medical specialty has grown, it has become more and difficult to have the same confidence in a broad arena of expertise. The *Homo sapien* has remained mostly the same, except for some minor changes and environmental influences. Yet the pressure, both medically and legally, to be right has heightened dramatically.

I see it everyday in my practice. Primary care doctors often refer patients to me, having already treated them on four or five occasions without avail. When I examine the patient, a number of options appear. Sometimes the treatment is in the ballpark but not aggressive enough, and other times it's totally wrong. I don't blame the doctor. The ones I find at fault are those who, for their own ego, never ask for outside guidance, which is a harmful trait. One of my primary care friends refers to himself as a master of referral, and that's how the world has evolved. Handle the things you can handle, and send the others for a second opinion. It's what is best for the patient.

Evelyn Simon, referred from her primary care doctor, was a sweet 80-year-old woman.

"I've had this rash on my face. My doctor said he wasn't sure what it was."

Evelyn had *Herpes zoster*, otherwise known as shingles. The left side of her face, including part of her nose, was crusted and irritated from the infection. The left corner of her mouth drooped down, resigned to its current affliction.

I started her on an anti-viral medicine and an oral steroid for pain. I also recommended she see an ophthalmologist to make sure she did not suffer any eye damage.

"I can't whistle," she said. "My face is all numb. And I just started to open and close my left eye."

"I'll see you again soon," I said, "I believe you'll get better every day. Don't worry."

Evelyn gave me a droopy smile, but a smile nonetheless. Given her hardy nature, I had a good feeling she would get better soon.

Ernie Bailey, my chronic psoriasis patient, came back in. I greeted him with a smile and a handshake. "Hello, Ernie."

"Listen, Doc," he starts, from his perch on the examining table (the only thing missing was a microphone and a bigger audience), "A woman has twins, and gives them up for adoption. One of them goes to a family in Egypt and is named Amal. The other goes to a family in Spain and they name him Juan. Years later Juan sends a picture of himself to his mom. Upon receiving the picture, she tells her husband that she wishes she also had a picture of Amal. Her husband tells her, 'Listen, honey, they're twins. If you've seen Juan, you've seen Amal!'"

"That's good, Ernie," I said. We always had time for his health problems, but he preferred to spend the time telling jokes. I think he had enough to deal with in his life, and by keeping us entertained, he could get "out of himself." I didn't complain. I always enjoyed his humor and kindness.

Linda Corvane sat down, and immediately spouted out words and more words.

"I was going to this primary care doctor, and I had just had surgery, and my surgeon told my primary care doctor to keep close watch on me; that I was borderline diabetic. So he treated me for a whole year with antibiotics and nerve drugs.

"And so finally I had red spots on my face and itchy spots, and I had sugar in my kidneys, and just about everything I think I had had sugar in it.

"And so I came out to see him, and I can't forget it. I thought, 'That doctor's kind of odd. Looks like he's wanting to shoot me. Get me out!'

"He said, 'Does your face stay that red all the time?' And I said, 'No.' And I was just thinking maybe it was because he was a new doctor; it was the first time I had seen him.

"So he checked me out and all. And I knew he kind of acted funny and all to be a new doctor. So he called me at the house – and these doctors don't usually call you at home. So he called me at the house. I saw him on Thursday. Friday, he called me. He says, 'I want you to go see your primary care doctor.' And I said, 'Well, Dr Silver was my doctor.'

"So I kept going to him, and I was so sick 'til I had to be led around the office back and forth. And I kept telling him, 'I'm going to the bathroom every 45 minutes. I'm not getting any sleep. I'm just dead on my feet.'

"And he wrote me a prescription for Xanax [Alprazolam] and Cipro [Ciprofloxacin], and I stayed on that for … well, until they brought in this other doctor. Because he called on Friday, and they had this doctor in there Monday, and he put me on the diabetic medicine and all.

"So things are still going, but I was blind for more than a year. And I went to this healing service. I was blind the 24th of November, and the 24th of December in '97, I went to this healing service, and I got my sight back. So these little dibs and dabs, you know, of things that are still going on.

"At the healing service, they just put their hands on my eyes and prayed for me. Well, he put his hands over my eyes, and I went out. And then two people picked me up, and he says, 'What do you see?' And he held his thumb up like that [demonstrating]. And he says, 'What do you see?'

"And I says, 'I see your thumb.' And I went out again, and I was out for about two hours.

"But anyway, I got my sight back Christmas of '97, and I was in Wal-Mart with my daughter and all of a sudden, you know, she says, 'Don't touch this.' I'm scared I'm going to fall down. And I kept telling her, 'Leave me alone.' I said, 'I see that man clear across to the wall over there.' You know, Wal-Mart is a good, wide store; and I see that man stacking dog food over there.

"I went off by myself. And this was a beautiful store I had all around me; it looked like God had opened up heaven.

"And I told the doctor about it last time I was out there, and he said, 'If you want to see something beautiful,' he said, 'come to my house when my three boys have gone through it.'

"But, you know, after being blind for more than a year and seeing everything all of a sudden, you know.... That's all I can think of."

She let out her breath, a deflated tire of talk, and was still for a moment. A wonderful, odd moment.

"You've had an amazing life," I said, feeling like I had been on an out-of-control boat that had just docked and I had finally stepped off on the shore. "Let's concentrate on your current problems, and we'll come up with some answers, OK?"

"Sure, Doctor," she said. "That sounds good to me."

After a few stops and starts, we eventually weaved together her story.

No matter what field of medicine you practice, it's a lot of work, and the story is often hard to get down. As with most challenging jobs, the work requires lots of patience. And here it is especially true – patience with patients. With patience stories get told, things get done, people get better.